HEALTH CARE TERMS
Healthy Communities Edition

Vergil N. Slee, MD
Debora A. Slee, JD
H. Joachim Schmidt, JD

Tringa Press
Saint Paul, Minnesota

© 1996 by Tringa Press

Tringa Press
P.O. Box 8181
St. Paul, MN 55108
612-222-7476
http://www.tringa.com

ISBN 0-9615255-7-6

Printed by Kaye's Printing in the United States of America on recycled paper.

99 98 97 96   9 8 7 6 5 4 3 2 1

Preface

What happened to health care reform? It's still here — more than ever. The failed 1993 drive in Congress to enact federal health care reform legislation had several results:

The majority of Congress acknowledged that prescribing a health care system for the entire country at the federal level was not a realistic goal. One size could not fit all, and probably no central body could create a system with the flexibility required to meet the unique needs of communities across the United States.

States were awakened to the issues involved in health care — cost, waste, equity, access, accountability, quality, prevention, and security — and many of them began to enact measures which would be helpful in solving some of the problems.

Then there came a growing conviction that even state-level solutions would not fit all local problems and needs.

Communities across the country began to struggle harder with their own most pressing problems — and in doing so they discovered unmet needs, unwarranted local program overlapping, and untapped local resources. They began to develop innovative and unique solutions.

Communities increasingly became convinced that the health *care* system should be renamed and also be redefined. It should be a *health* system concerned about the health of all, rather than a care system responsible only for the persons who present themselves.

Hospitals in increasing numbers adopted this conviction and modified their mission statements to show responsibility for the health of the entire community. This is a major change of focus: outreach is added to response.

Thus the nascent Healthy Communities movement emerged and took on a life of its own. Health care reform at the local level began growing strong.

Nonetheless, despite the growing trend toward solving health and health care problems at the community level, there clearly are "higher level" legislative and regulatory steps which would facilitate the healthy communities movement. Among them:

- revision of anti-trust statutes which prevent cooperation and collaboration among providers;

- tort reform, to reduce insurance costs, relieve fear, and diminish defensive medicine;

- modification of regulations of granting agencies which interfere with local collaboration and sharing of resources;

- elimination of micromanagement of federal and state programs;

- enactment of insurance regulations which provide portability of benefits, access for those with pre-existing conditions, and community rating.

This book is aimed at helping community leaders — both professional and nonprofessional — gain the understanding of concepts and terminology in health care needed to work collaboratively to find solutions to build healthy communities.

Introduction

What is Health Care Reform?

"Health care reform" includes all the efforts to solve the problems of:

COST: Costs of health care are seen as too high and still rising. The United States spends a much larger share of the gross domestic product on health care than any other country and, critics say, our health doesn't reflect the difference. Health care costs, which must be covered by the prices of our products and our taxes, are seen as a major reason that the United States is losing its competitive position in the world market.

WASTE: The media are full of stories about waste, unnecessary care, and fraud. Even if not all of this attention is warranted, it provides fuel for the reform movement.

EQUITY: Inequities among regions of the country, between rural and urban settings, among ethnic groups, and among socioeconomic groups, in access to and quality of both preventive and curative services, are widely reported.

ACCESS: There is increasing concern not only with access in its traditional meaning, having to do with the ability of the individual to physically get to and utilize health care facilities, but also with "access" meaning eligibility for (access to) insurance benefits. A person whose income is too high to qualify for Medicaid in a given state, for example, does not have access to Medicaid benefits. People with preexisting medical conditions, who are poor risks, or who cannot afford insurance often have no coverage at all.

ACCOUNTABILITY: Society is demanding that health care providers show evidence as to the quality of care they deliver, and also their stewardship of resources.

QUALITY: Care is alleged to be of variable quality from place to place and from provider to provider. And there are charges and fears that cost containment is tantamount to lowering quality.

PREVENTION: There is a growing recognition that prevention, of illnesses and injuries, as well as of the progression of illness, saves money. Yet preventive services are absent from most health insurance policies and many health care plans.

SECURITY: People lose their health insurance when they change jobs, so they are sometimes "locked in" to their employment. Some cannot obtain health insurance. And they are concerned that health care will destroy them financially. A stated goal of health care reform is that people will never lose their insurance, and that health care will not bankrupt individuals.

Why is it Happening Now?

In addition to the above concerns to the American people, other changes are occurring today in our society at the personal level which provide an impetus to make fundamental changes in our health care system. These are "paradigm shifts" in the way an increasing number of people think about being and staying healthy, and about their relationships with their health care providers. Several significant shifts are:

1. From the view that health care providers are there to provide "health care," to the view that "health" rather than "health care" is their goal.

2. From the view that knowledge processing is limited to the human mind, plus "paper and pencil," to the view that knowledge processing can be successfully extended through the use of computer technology.

3. From the view that the physician should retain the "paternal" role of caring and making decisions for the patient, to the view that empowered and enabled patients are competent to collaborate in their own health care and that, in fact, many wish to and can direct their own care.

4. From the view that the government is responsible for the health of the community, to the view that the community itself is responsible.

About the Authors

Vergil N. Slee, MD, MPH, is Chairman of the Board of the Health Commons Institute and President Emeritus of the Commission on Professional and Hospital Activities (CPHA). He pioneered the Professional Activity Study (PAS) and founded CPHA, and was president of the Council on Clinical Classifications which, with the U.S. National Center for Health Statistics, created the *Clinical Modification* of the *International Classification of Diseases, Ninth Revision (ICD-9-CM)*. Dr. Slee has served for over thirty years as a member of the faculty of Estes Park Institute (EPI), which presents national conferences for hospital trustees, administrators, medical staff officers, physicians, and community representatives, on emerging health care issues. He is a Fellow of the American College of Physicians, a Fellow of the American Public Health Association, and an Honorary Fellow of the American College of Healthcare Executives.

Debora A. Slee, JD, is an attorney and writer with experience in managed care organization and licensure, health care law, and quality management. She is contributing author to *The Law of Hospital and Health Care Administration, Second Edition*, by Arthur F. Southwick, and coauthor of *Health Care Terms, Second Edition*.

H. Joachim Schmidt, JD, is a retired farmer and lawyer who currently amuses himself by riding on the wave of information technology. A veteran software applications engineer, he is now specializing in infoweaving — making information more accessible by use of new electronic tools like hypertext and multimedia.

A

AAPCC   See *Average Adjusted Per Capita Cost.*

AARP   See *American Association of Retired Persons.*

abuse (health care)   The improper or excessive use of health care products and services. Abuse may result from excessive (unnecessary) use of diagnostic tests, unnecessary surgical and other procedures, and so forth. Abuse may be either intentional or unintentional, and may or may not be illegal.

The laws governing Medicare, for example, make certain referral arrangements illegal because they create opportunity for abuse, even though there may be no actual abuse or intent to abuse. See *fraud and abuse.*

accelerated death benefit   An amount paid to an individual, under a life insurance contract, when that individual has been diagnosed with a specific medical condition (generally a terminal illness). After that person's death, the balance is paid to the beneficiary just like any other life insurance.

access (physical)   Physical access. Access ordinarily means the ability of patients to physically get to (or into) health care. Facilities and resources must be located where they can be reached, and they must be designed so that handicapped persons may enter, i.e, "barrier-free access".

access (to health care)   The ability to obtain health care. Access includes available physicians and facilities, transportation, acceptance by the facility, and means of payment. "Access" is often used specifically to mean eligibility for (access to) insurance benefits, since lack of insurance can be a formidable barrier to receiving health care. Individuals who are above a given state's definition of the poverty level for qualification for Medicaid are said to be denied access. In 1990, for example, when the federal poverty threshold was $13,356, access was very different in a state which had its Medicaid threshold at $3,000 (family income above this amount disqualifies the family for Medicaid) than in a state where the threshold was $10,000. Thus an unemployed or employed low income person who cannot be insured through an employer might not qualify for public assistance, either.

accountability   The obligation to provide, to all concerned, the evidence needed to: (1) establish confidence that the task or duty for which one is responsible is being or has been performed; and (2) describe the manner in which that task is being or has been carried out. When accountability has been fulfilled, the authority which delegated the responsibility can be satisfied by evidence (rather than simply assertion) that the duties or tasks which have been delegated are being or have been adequately performed.

Accountability must be defined in conjunction with responsibility. An individual or organization has responsibility (that is to say, an obligation) because some individual or body with authority has granted or delegated that responsibility. Failure to carry out the responsibility carries with it liability. A responsible party is entitled to delegate duties, that is, to get help in carrying out the obligation, but not to delegate the responsibility itself. The responsible party, therefore, must have reasonable ground on which he can render account (be accountable) for the duties which have been delegated. So the delegation of duties, as a matter of law, carries with it the requirement of accountability to the source of the delegation of the duties.

A hospital, for example, is delegated certain duties by "society," by government. For this purpose, the hospital's responsibility is accepted and held by its governing body. The governing body must render account for its performance (it holds accountability) to society, through specific reporting mechanisms, voluntary efforts to provide society evidence of its performance, and defending itself against liability suits. In turn the governing body delegates tasks to the chief executive officer (CEO) and demands accounting from that individual; the CEO, in turn, delegates tasks to departmental heads and demands accountability from them.

Similarly, the governing body gives the medical staff duties, for example, with respect to the credentialing of applicants for medical staff membership. The medical staff incurs, along with the duty, the obligation of accountability—it must provide the evidence needed to establish the governing body's confidence that it, the medical staff, has indeed performed the task, and the evidence must be presented in enough detail to permit the governing body to assess the quality of performance of the duty.

accountable health partnership (AHP) See *accountable health plan.*

accountable health plan (AHP) A proposed form of health care plan which would be accountable for meeting certain federal requirements for providing certain standardized health services. Synonym(s): accountable health partnership (AHP), approved health plan (AHP).

accreditation A process of: (1) evaluation of an institution or education program to determine whether it meets the standards set up by an accrediting body, and (2) if the institution or program meets the standards, granting recognition of the fact. Accreditation is a process performed by a non-governmental agency at the request of the institution or education program. Although governmental agencies carry out evaluation and recognition processes on a mandatory basis for licensure purposes, these processes are not accreditation.

Health care institutions are accredited by the Joint Commission on Accreditation of Healthcare Organizations (JCAHO) in the United States and by the Canadian Council on Health Facilities Accreditation (CCHFA) in Canada. Health care education programs are accredited by other bodies.

actuary A mathematician who specializes in estimating risks, rates, premiums, and other factors for insurance companies.

acuity Acuteness, as of an illness. The term is used a great deal in reference to nursing needs and demands for other health care resources: the greater the acuity, the more nursing care or other services are needed.

Adjusted Community Rate (ACR)   A term used by HCFA in its Medicare risk contracts with HMO/CMPs to mean the premium the HMO would charge for providing exactly the same Medicare-covered benefits to a community rated group, adjusted to allow for the greater intensity and frequency of utilization by Medicare recipients. See also *community rating* and *adjusted community rating,* under *rating.*

administrative law   The body of law which governs the powers of administrative agencies, the process of agency decision-making, and the procedures by which a party can challenge an adverse decision of an agency.

admitting privileges   See *privileges.*

adult day health services   Medical and other health care services provided to patients whose condition permits them to return home or to another facility at night. When such care is regularly scheduled, it may be termed partial hospitalization. Synonym(s): day health care services.

advance directive   A statement executed by a person while of sound mind as to that person's wishes about the use of medical interventions for him or her self in case of the loss of his or her own decision-making capacity. A number of forms of advance directives have been proposed and are used; some are described below. See also *Patient Self-Determination Act (PSDA).*

durable power of attorney   A power of attorney which remains (or becomes) effective when the principal becomes incompetent to act for herself. It should be noted that in most states, even an agent with a durable power of attorney cannot make medical treatment decisions for an incompetent patient, unless state law provides that she can or a court has given her specific authority.

health care proxy   A document which authorizes a designated person (who is also called a "proxy") to make health care decisions in the event that the signer is incapable of making those decisions. State law governs whether such a document is valid, how it must be created, and to what extent the proxy is authorized to make health care decisions. For example, a proxy may not be able to consent to electroconvulsive therapy or sterilization.

instructional advance directive (IAD)   An advance directive in which an attempt is made to allow the person executing the directive to record quite specifically those interventions which are not to be attempted in case of the loss of the person's own decision-making capacity.

The Medical Directive   An instructional advance directive document published in the New England Journal of Medicine in 1989 which has been made available to the lay public. The Medical Directive describes four clinical scenarios, each of which affects the patient's own decision-making capacity, and then lists a series of medical diagnostic or therapeutic interventions. The person who completes the document checks off whether he would choose the interventions in the case of each of the scenarios. The completed document is interpreted as an advance directive for the person who completes it.

value history   A type of instructional advance directive which attempts to elicit the attitudes and personal values of an individual so that someone reading the history would be able to deduct the decisions with regard to medical care which one could expect the individual completing the value history to make. The value history would be used to guide others in determining the care an individual would like to have rendered in case the individual lost his or her own decision-making capacity.

living will   A will concerning the life of the individual executing the will, in contrast with the usual "last will and testament" in which the subject matter is the disposition of property (this could be thought of as a "property will") and custody of minor children. In many states, individuals may execute "living wills" concerning the circumstances under which they wish to refuse, or discontinue the use of, life-support measures administered to themselves should they become incompetent. Living will statutes (also known as right to die laws or natural death acts) govern the execution and enforcement procedures for living wills. At least one state (New Hampshire) calls the living will a "terminal care document."

The "life-sustaining procedures act," proposed by the National Conference of Commissioners on Uniform State Laws, suggests the following language for a living will: "If I should have an incurable or irreversible condition that will cause my death within a relatively short time, and if I am unable to make decisions regarding my medical treatment, I direct my attending physician to withhold or withdraw procedures that merely prolong the dying process and are not necessary to my comfort or to alleviate pain."

adverse selection   A situation in which patients with greater than average need for medical and hospital care enroll in a prepaid health plan in greater numbers than they occur in a cross-section of the population. A plan which somehow encouraged or allowed people to sign up when they were already ill would suffer from adverse selection.

advocacy   Attempting to persuade others of the rightness of a cause, or of a point of view on an issue. Such educational efforts—for example, health education—are increasingly undertaken by hospitals and other nonprofit organizations, but if they are addressed at passing or defeating legislation, they may be classified as lobbying and therefore endanger the organization's tax-exempt status.

affiliation   Any one of a number of arrangements among providers outlining their relationships and their individual responsibilities. The relationships are contained in documents which range from broad letters of intent to detailed contracts. In the past, such arrangements were often called alliances, but this term was preempted in the health care reform movement by proposals for specific organizations labelled "health care alliances," which were often referred to merely as "alliances."

agency (administrative)   Administrative agency. A part of state or federal government, created by the legislature, which has specific administrative duties and functions, often including regulation of a profession or industry. A state board of medical examiners, for example, is an administrative agency. There is a body of law (administrative law) which governs the powers of administrative agencies, the process of agency decision-making, and the procedures by which a party dissatisfied with a decision of an agency can challenge it. Ordinarily, any person who wishes to contest an administrative agency decision must go through all of the channels of appeal within the agency before challenging the decision in the courts.

agency (legal) A legal relationship in which one person acts on behalf of another. A written agency agreement is called a power of attorney.

agency (organization) An organization set up to carry out services such as home health care, "meals on wheels," or registration of tumor patients. In this usage, the agency may be part of either the public sector or the private sector. If the agency is private, it may be either nonprofit or for-profit.

Agency for Health Care Policy and Research (AHCPR) A component of the Public Health Service (PHS), which is in turn a component of the Department of Health and Human Services (DHHS). Among its functions is the dissemination of information about the assessment of health technology. See *Office of Health Technology Assessment (OHTA)*.

agent (facilitator) An instrument or means by which something is done. Often used to describe a person working within an organization:

change agent A person whose efforts, by design or not, facilitate change in an organization. Such a person may not even be aware of causing change.

energy agent A term which more accurately describes the role of an individual who provides leadership, from within the organization or outside it, to enhance the productivity and satisfaction of individuals. For many years the emphasis has been on "change agents"; however, at least as much effort must be employed for entropy prevention as for change. The term "energy agent" covers both of these tasks of management (as well as individuals who are effective in creating and maintaining an organization's enthusiasm and productivity).

Aid to Families with Dependent Children (ADC, AFDC) A federally financed program for single-parent families, designed to provide welfare for single parents who cannot, without this assistance, take proper care of the children.

all-payer plan A payment policy under which the same payment method is applied to patients of all payers. Today, the term "all-payer plan" really means applying the prospective payment system (PPS) to all patients, rather than Medicare patients only. (Medicare patients are the only patients to which the PPS applies under the present federal regulations.)

alliance In common usage, any one of a variety of collaborative arrangements among individuals or institutions. In the past, hospitals have formed alliances or affiliations, for example, between those furnishing primary, secondary, and tertiary care.

allied health professional A person who is not a physician, nurse, or pharmacist, and who works in the health field. An allied health professional may, for example, be a dietitian, an emergency medical technician, or an aide. Allied health professionals are sometimes called paraprofessionals or paramedical personnel. There are some 26 allied health professions for which educational standards have been developed.

allopathy

For a list of occupations for which programs have been accredited by the Committee on Allied Health Education and Accreditation (CAHEA), see that listing. Synonym(s): allied health personnel.

allopathy See *medicine (system)*.

Alpha Center A non-profit, private research organization focusing on health care financing and organizational issues. The Alpha Center also conducts a health care program for the uninsured in conjunction with the Robert Wood Johnson Foundation.

alternative delivery and financing system (ADFS) A general term which covers any kind of alternative organizational arrangement for the delivery of health care, such as a health maintenance organization (HMO), in which payment for physician services is other than fee-for-service (FFS). Thus, an ADFS is a combination of an alternative delivery system (ADS) and an alternative financing system (AFS).

alternative delivery system (ADS) (care) An alternative to traditional inpatient care, such as substitution of ambulatory care, home health care, hospice, or ambulatory surgery (same-day surgery). Synonym(s): alternative delivery mode.

alternative delivery system (ADS) (organization) An alternative to the traditional arrangements of health care providers into solo practice or group practice. Examples include the independent physician association (IPA), preferred provider organization (PPO), health maintenance organization (HMO), and health care organization (HCO). The method of purchase of service or payment of physicians (fee-for-service (FFS) or capitation, for example) does not govern the term in this usage.

alternative dispute resolution (ADR) Methods of settling claims and disagreements other than by the traditional method—a lawsuit.

administrative determination of fault (ADF) A proposed method of alternative dispute resolution combining features of a compensation fund and arbitration. Claims would be filed with a designated agency which would determine whether or not there were negligence and, if there were, the claimant would be paid from a fund. Provision would be made for administrative appeal.

arbitration When used as a method of alternative dispute resolution, providers and patients would agree in advance to have any disputes handled by arbitration rather than going to court.

compensation fund A fund into which insurers, practitioners, and facilities would deposit moneys to be used to compensate anyone "injured in the course of receiving health care services, regardless of whether the provider or professional was negligent."

early offer A form of alternative dispute resolution (ADR) in which the practitioner or provider could, in cases of injury, make an offer which, if accepted, would preclude certain court actions and result in prompt payment for costs (but not for pain and suffering). See also *patients' compensation* under *compensation*.

alternative financing system (AFS) An alternative to the fee-for-service (FFS) payment system, such as a health care organization (HCO), health maintenance organization (HMO), or competitive medical plan (CMP) in which some other mechanism, usually capitation, is the method of payment to the organization and sometimes to the physician.

alternative medicine Unconventional therapies, such as massage, biofeedback, herbal remedies, and acupuncture. There appears to be consensus that these therapies should be evaluated; contention arises from insistence by physicians that the therapies should be judged by the same research standards as are other therapies, while their advocates resist this rigid protocol. In Europe, and increasingly in the United States, the term "complementary medicine", is used for alternative medicine, since its techniques are usually not replacements for other therapies, but rather are additional treatment resources. A 1992 report to the National Institutes of Health, Alternative Medicine: Expanding Medical Horizons, classifies alternative medicine methods into 7 categories: mind-body interventions; bioelectromagnetics applications in medicine; alternative systems of medical practice; manual healing methods; pharmacological and biological treatments; herbal medicine; and diet and nutrition in the prevention and treatment of chronic diseases.

ambulatory A term which specifically means "able to walk," but which in health care refers to a person who is not bedridden. Thus a person who requires a wheel chair is ambulatory, and can come in for treatment and return home.

ambulatory care Care provided to a patient without hospitalization.

Ambulatory Patient Group (APG) A way of classifying hospital outpatient procedures for reimbursement purposes that is similar to the DRG system for inpatient services. Ambulatory patients are grouped according to clinical characteristics, resource use, and costs. 3M Health Information Systems developed the system for HCFA.

American Association for Medical Systems and Informatics (AAMSI) A national organization interested in the application of computers to medical problems.

American Association of Retired Persons (AARP) An organization often referred to in current health care literature (sometimes only by its acronym) because of its intense activity in regard to health legislation, health care financing, access, and quality.

American Health Information Management Association (AHIMA) The national association of health information management professionals. Operates a publishing business, manages professional practice, library, and certification services, and accredits educational programs. AHIMA conducts exams and provides certification for Registered Record Administrators (RRAs) and Accredited Record Administrators (ARTs). Formerly the American Medical Records Association (AMRA)

American Hospital System Although this term is often used, there really is no such thing as the "American Hospital System," except that the nation's hospitals and other health care facilities, along with health professionals and allied health professionals, do make up an informal network across the country through which care is provided. The "American Hospital System" simply means what actually exists—community hospitals, university hospitals, nonprofit hospitals, investor-owned hospitals, government hospitals, and the like.

American Public Health Association (APHA)   The national association which embraces all public health professionals.

American Society for Testing and Materials (ASTM)   An organization originally concerned with developing standards for and testing industrial materials, but which has more recently been doing similar work with computer systems, many of them in the medical field.

Americans with Disabilities Act (ADA)   A federal law which prohibits discrimination against persons with physical or mental disabilities by private sector service providers, employers, and state and local governments. The law requires reasonable accommodation and equal opportunity for persons with disabilities. It became effective in 1992.

ancillary personnel   Personnel other than physicians and nurses.

ancillary services   Hospital services other than room and board. In a hospital, nursing services are included as part of "room and board"; since normal nursing services are not billed for separately, they are not ancillary services.
    The Oregon plan defines ancillary services as those services which are considered to be integral to successful treatment of a condition. Examples given are hospital services, laboratory services, radiation therapy, prescription drugs, medical transportation, rehabilitation, maternity case management, and hospice services.

anhedonia   The absence of fun.

Annotated ICD-9-CM   A version of the International Classification of Diseases, Ninth Revision, Clinical Modification (ICD-9-CM) which is color-coded to alert users to reimbursement-related issues. It is published by the Commission on Professional and Hospital Activities (CPHA).

anti-dumping law   A law which prohibits the transfer or discharge of patients for financial rather than medical reasons. See *dumping* and *Consolidated Omnibus Budget Reconciliation Act of 1985 (COBRA)*.

antikickback law   Sometimes used to refer to the Medicare fraud and abuse laws, which prohibit, among other things, paying or receiving "kickbacks" for referral of Medicare patients. See *fraud and abuse*.

antitrust   That branch of law which seeks to prevent monopolies and unfair competition. A "trust" was originally a combination of several corporations (each maintaining its separate identity) to eliminate competition, control prices, and the like. The term "antitrust" now broadly covers any activity (or conspiracy) to eliminate competition and control the marketplace. It includes actions which unreasonably restrain trade. Such activities are illegal, and severe penalties are imposed by antitrust laws. For example, the trust may be broken up, and anyone who suffers injury to his business or property as a result of the combination or conspiracy may collect treble damages. Federal antitrust laws (principally the Sherman Act of 1890, the Clayton Act of 1914, and the Federal Trade Commission Act of 1914) apply to companies doing business in interstate commerce. Many states also have antitrust laws.

Antitrust problems may arise for hospitals when they place limitations on medical staff membership, for example, or when several hospitals seek to combine services. Careful legal guidance is required in any area in which a hospital's actions may affect competition or regulate prices.

Antitrust issues are of concern in health care reform because of the fear that innovative approaches to health care organization and delivery of service may be deemed to be in violation of the antitrust regulations. Serious consideration is being given to amending the laws or providing for exceptions in order to stimulate and facilitate experimentation, and avoid unnecessary duplication of services.

any willing provider   A law in some states which requires a managed care organization, such as an HMO, to grant participation to any provider who is legally qualified as a practitioner and who is willing to become a member of the organization. Such laws are enacted to protect the patient's freedom of choice. However they often interfere seriously with the efforts ot the managed care organization to achieve high quality and efficiency by limiting its provider network to caregivers with the best performance records, to hospitals in convenient geographic locations, and to selected pharmacies.

APG   See *Ambulatory Patient Group*

appropriateness   A term used in connection with review of care to indicate whether the measures taken were proper under the circumstances, and whether it would have been proper to have taken other measures under the circumstances.

APR   See *Average Payment Rate.*

area wage adjustment   A component of the payment formula under the prospective payment system (PPS) to allow for differences in wage scales in different parts of the country.

artificial intelligence (AI)   A term used to describe a type of system in which the computer appears to be "thinking," and thus exhibits intelligence. Although the system appears to "think," it really does not; rather, it has been given a number of "rules" to follow. A simple example would be a billing system which follows the rule: if there has been no payment within 30 days, send letter "A"; if there has been no payment within 60 days, send letter "B." Another example would be a program which looks up "unfamiliar" words (those not in its memory): if the word is a synonym for or similar to a word to which the system should respond and take action, it will either go ahead with the action or ask a human to confirm its "decision." There is some tendency for computer salespeople to overuse the term "artificial intelligence" to gain a sales advantage; this leads the customer to believe that AI systems are invariably better for every task than other systems.

artificial neural system   See *neurocomputer* under *computer.*

asset   An object (property or money, for example), a right (to royalties, for example), or a claim (a title to a debt, for example) which its owners consider to be of benefit to them. Assets in hospitals include property and equipment (which may have less value than their original cost because of depreciation), investments, accounts receivable (claims to money owed to the institution), and the other items which are listed as "assets" on the balance sheet of the institution.

assignment (of benefits)   A voluntary decision by the beneficiary to have insurance benefits paid directly to the provider rather than to the beneficiary him or herself. The act requires the signing of a form for the purpose. The provider is not obligated to accept an assignment of benefits; it may refuse and instead require the beneficiary to handle the collection procedure. Conversely, the provider may insist on assignment in order to protect its revenue; if the provider accepts the assignment, it ordinarily assumes responsibility for the collection paperwork.

audit   A term which usually means a financial audit, in which the organization's financial statement, and the degree to which the statement reflects the actual affairs of the organization, are examined. An audit also includes a review of the procedures used to keep records, prevent losses of funds and equipment, and the like. An audit may be an internal audit or an external audit. When the term is used without a modifier, "audit" refers to an external audit by a public accountant (PA).

An audit may also made of the organization's compliance with its own policies and with grant and contract obligations, of its management efficiency, or of its quality management.

external audit   An audit carried out by an independent public accountant. "Independent" means that the auditor is not an employee of the audited organization, and does not have certain other forbidden connections with the organization.

internal audit   An administrative process carried out in organizations, by the organization's own employees, in an effort to determine the extent to which the organization's internal operations conform with its own intended procedures and practices. When a similar review is done by an outside group, it is called an external audit.

patient care audit (PCA)   The preferred term for the process also called "medical audit" or "medical care evaluation study." A patient care audit is a retrospective review of the quality of care of a group of patients, ordinarily a group with the same diagnosis or therapy. The review is based on medical records, and matches the care against standards of care. "Patient care audit" is the preferred term because it indicates that the focus of the study is the care received by the group of patients, rather than the performance of physicians, nurses, or other caregivers.

quality management audit   An audit of the quality management of an institution, similar in intent and conduct to a fiscal audit, but addressed at the quality function rather than the fiscal function.

auxiliary   Providing help.

hospital auxiliary   A organization, whose membership is from the community, whose purpose is to assist the hospital. Often called simply the auxiliary.

average adjusted per capita cost (AAPCC)   A dollar amount arrived at by actuarial projection, which is meant to represent the average annual cost for a Medicare beneficiary in a particular geographic area. The AAPCC is the basis of the government's payment to HMOs and other risk-based providers for Medicare beneficiaries. The government pays the HMO 95 percent of the AAPCC. If the medicare beneficiaries are relatively healthy in a particular region, the 95 percent capitated payment results in the government paying more than if the same beneficiaries were enrolled in a fee-for-service plan. This payment method therefore has a built-in incentive for HMOs to attempt to enroll only the healthier Medicare beneficiaries (see *cherry picking*).

The government uses 1 of 122 possible monthly capitation amounts (rate cells) using five variables: age, gender, Medicaid eligibility, institutional status, and whether a person has both parts of Medicare (A & B). The AAPCC values are adjusted annually.

Average Payment Rate (APR)   The limit that HCFA may pay to a health maintenance organization (HMO) or competitive medical plan (CMP) for Medicare services under a risk contract. The APR is calculated for a particular geographic area, then adjusted according to the projected makeup of the HMO or CMP's Medicare enrollment. See also *adjusted average per capita cost* (AAPCC) and *adjusted community rate* (ACR).

B

balance billing   The practice of physicians to charge a patient the balance of charges when the patient's insurance (or other third party payer) will not pay the entire charge. For example, when Medicare will pay the physician only 80% of her or his usual fee for a given service, the physician sometimes "balance bills" the patient, who then has to pay the balance. A practitioner who has agreed to accept assignment as payment in full cannot balance bill the patient. See also *assignment (of benefits)* and *mandatory assignment*.

Federal legislation   (OBRA) in 1989 limited the amount a physician could balance bill to 115% of Medicare's approved rates for nonparticipating physicians. About 90% of physicians are participating, and thus must accept the amount Medicare pays them, and Medicare pays them faster, and 5% more, than it pays nonparticipating physicians. Since October 1994, the Health Care Financing Administration (HCFA) has been required to monitor "excess billing" by nonparticipating physicians, and can now refunds or credits from physicians who bill excessive amounts.

balance sheet   One of the two standard components of a financial statement, on which are shown the assets (what is owned) and the liabilities (what is owed) by the organization (see *liability (financial)*). An organization is most unlikely to find the assets and the liabilities exactly equal, so a third category of entry makes the sheet "balance": a line entitled "profit" or "loss." When assets exceed liabilities, the line shows a profit; when liabilities exceed assets, the line shows a loss. Since most hospitals are nonprofit, a line called "profit" would be inappropriate (although even a hospital could not survive if, over time, it owed more than it owned). Thus, most nonprofit organizations long ago abandoned the term "profit" and in its place adopted a euphemism such as "fund balance." A profit, then, would be called a "positive fund balance"; a loss would be called a "negative fund balance."

The other standard component of a financial statement is an income and expense statement (also called a profit and loss statement or operating statement).

bandwidth   A term coined in the 1930's to describe a range within a band of wavelengths of the radio frequency type. Its common usage today refers to the raw carrying capacity of a transmission medium, such as copper wires, fiber-optic cable, or satellite links. The greater the bandwidth, the more information can be transmitted. Telephones which also transmit the live picture of the persons speaking require much greater bandwidth than those transmitting the voice alone.

The implication for health care is the limitation on what kinds of information may be shared remotely. Transmitting a detailed x-ray picture to a distant site likely requires significantly greater bandwidth than all the *text* in a patient's medical record, for instance. The solution, of course, is to increase the transmission medium's bandwidth. A single fiber optic cable, for example, can carry the same number of telephone conversations as 3,200 copper wires. Increasing bandwidth is usually more of a political and economic issue than a technical one.

bar code system   A machine-readable coding system which uses a pattern of bars and empty spaces to convey a specific meaning. The system is commonly encountered in grocery stores and other retail establishments, where the bar code is read with a scanning device. The system usually calculates the bill, corrects the inventory of the item, and carries out other management and accounting functions. Bar codes are being standardized in the hospital industry for such purposes as recording the receipt of materials and supplies purchased by the hospital, maintaining their inventory, and making charges for them. Other hospital applications include recording services (such as in the laboratory or emergency department), posting the charges to the patient bills and to the appropriate revenue and expense accounts, and inventory control. When so used, the bar code is an input device for a point of sale system. An example of bar coding can be found on the back cover of this book, on which this book's ISBN number is displayed in both human-readable and machine-readable bar code formats.

bare-bones health plan   A no-frills health care plan or health care insurance policy with limited coverage, large deductibles and copayments, and low policy limits. Designed to be affordable to small businesses.

base (rate)   A statistical term referring to the "per" number in a given rate. A ratio or proportion is often expressed as a percentage (per 100), but it may also be expressed per 1,000, per 10,000, per 100,000, or even per million. These "per" numbers are called the "base." Thus a percentage is said to have 100 as the base. The base chosen is usually large enough to ensure that the rate will be expressed in whole numbers; the more rare the event, the larger the base used. For example, a death rate of 7 per 10,000 simply is easier to understand than a rate of 0.07 percent, although both actually give the same information.

base (measure) A reference quantity or reference time, often a given year. For example, the data used in calculating a consumer price index (CPI) include base prices, which are prices found in the year chosen as the base.

base unit A procedure or service used in developing a relative value scale (RVS). See *relative value scale (RVS)*.

base year Medicare costs A hospital's costs for the base year from which computations are made in the Medicare payment formula. The base year is, by definition, always several years behind the present, and its costs are those as determined according to the federal regulations for cost allocations.

bed A bed for an inpatient in a hospital or other health care facility.

bed capacity The number of patients a hospital can hold. A hospital may have different bed capacity figures depending on whether one refers to its constructed beds, its licensed beds, or its regularly maintained beds. Thus, a statement of capacity should always tell which is intended. It is possible, though, that bed capacity figures may all be the same for a given hospital at a given moment.

constructed beds The number of beds the hospital was built to accommodate.

licensed beds The number of beds which the state licensing agency authorizes the hospital to operate on a regular basis.

regularly maintained beds The number of beds a hospital has set up for daily operation (in units of the hospital in use and staffed) on a regular basis. This number may change from time to time. It would ordinarily be a number smaller than the number of licensed beds or the number of constructed beds. The count is usually expressed in three segments: for adult inpatients, pediatric patients, and newborns. See *bed count*.

bed conversion The reassignment of beds by the hospital from one use to another, for example, the reassignment of beds from acute care to long-term care use. When such a conversion is done in both directions (when it is, depending on changing circumstances, reversible) the beds are usually called swing beds. In some states, certain types of conversion must be permanent and can only be made with permission of the state licensing authority.

bed count The number of beds a hospital maintains regularly for the use of inpatients.

bed day A way to measure the utilization of hospital inpatient facilities.

available bed days The number of bed days which the hospital is set up to provide in a given time period. It is computed by multiplying the number of regularly maintained beds (see *bed capacity*) by the number of days in the time period. Available bed days are ordinarily expressed in three segments: available adult inpatient service days; available newborn bed days; and available pediatric (child) inpatient bed days. See also *bed* and *bed count*.

occupied bed day   The period of time between the taking of the hospital census on two successive days (the census is taken at the same hour each day). In counting the length of stay (LOS) of a patient, "the day of admission is an occupied bed day, the day of discharge is not." Application of this rule gives one day of stay to a patient who is admitted and discharged during a single occupied bed day.

bed pan mutual   A slang term for a physician-owned professional liability insurance company.

bed turnover rate   See *rate (ratio)*.

behavior offset   A overall percentage decrease in physician fees to be paid by Medicare during the period of transition to the resource based relative value scale (RBRVS). The assumption was made by the Health Care Financing Administration (HCFA) that physicians would attempt to adjust to the RBRVS (which will reduce physician fees for certain services) by increasing their volume of services, i.e., by changing their behavior. Thus the fee reduction to counter this and keep the total Medicare spending for physician services from increasing was termed by HCFA a "behavior offset." The process of adopting the RBRVS also had a "volume adjustment" aimed at the same goal, and a great deal of opposition developed in Congress as well as among physicians against the additional behavior offset.

benchmark   The performance, with respect to a given attribute, of an organization or individual whose performance is considered to be the goal of others. In the context of health care reform, benchmark performance would be that which delivers the best combination of results and cost; i.e., the "best" possible outcome may cost so much that it cannot be taken as a benchmark.

benchmarking   A system whereby health care assessment undertakes to measure its performance against "best practice" standards. Best practice standards can reflect: (1) Evidence-based medical practice. This is practice supported by current investigative studies of like patient populations. (2) Knowledge-based systems. Explicit in benchmarking is movement away from anecdotal and single-practitioner experience based practice: "I had a patient once who . . . "

beneficiary   The person entitled to benefits from insurance or some other health care financing program, such as Medicare—the person "insured" as contrasted with the owner of the policy, for example.

benefit package   The array or set of benefits (services covered) included in or provided by a given insurance "policy." The term is widely heard in the health care reform discussions; one does not hear it used in connection with automobile insurance, for example.

basic benefit package   A standard benefit package which contains the services which must be the *least* which can be provided to any insured individual. Such a package would be the "floor" under the health benefits given to any individual. States, insurance companies, employers, or others could offer or provide additional benefits at their discretion. Health care reform discussions assume the existence of such a package. Also called "core benefit package" or "benchmark benefit package."

benchmark benefit package   See *basic benefit package.*

core benefit package   See *basic benefit package.*

defined benefit package   See *standard benefit package.*

Medicare benefit package   The federal government defines a basic benefit package for Medicare beneficiaries at the federal level for those for whom it provides coverage, and Medicare benefits are thus uniform throughout the country. Medicaid benefit packages, on the other hand, are determined by each state.

standard benefit package   A uniform (usually mandated) package of health insurance or health plan benefits. The purposes of standard benefit packages are to permit purchasers to compare among plans as to price and to prevent risk selection by the plans. For true plan comparison, there must also be standard definitions of benefits.

supplemental benefit package   Any array or set of benefits to be added to the basic benefit package. Definition or standardization of the contents of the package is not implied in the term, except in the case of the Medicare supplemental insurance packages.

uniform benefit package   See *standard benefit package.*

Uniform Effective Health Benefits (UEHB)   A term employed by the Jackson Hole Group meaning a "list of effective and appropriate health care services that will constitute the national standard for health care every American will be eligible to receive under the managed competition proposal."

benefits   The money, care, or other services to which an individual is entitled by virtue of insurance. In health care insurance, there are two basic kinds of benefits, indemnity benefits and service benefits.

indemnity benefits   Insurance benefits provided in cash to the beneficiary rather than in services. Indemnity benefits are usual with commercial insurance. Payment may go directly to the provider, or to reimburse the beneficiary.

service benefits   Insurance benefits which are the health care services themselves, rather than money. Service benefits are traditional with Blue Cross/Blue Shield (BC/BS) and Medicare. In fact, the unique nature of service benefits led to special legislation for the Blue Cross and Blue Shield plans when they were established, and the granting of their original nonprofit charters.

bereavement care   Care which assists with the physical, emotional, spiritual, psychological, social, financial, and legal needs of the survivor(s) of a person who has died.

bill   A statement from the provider of the charges for services, drugs, appliances, use of facilities, and other items for a given patient's care, for example, for an emergency department admission or an inpatient episode of care.

billing   Notifying patients or their third party payers of the charges for services rendered, along with the amount due.

combined billing   A billing in which the hospital and physician services and their charges are not separately identified. Certain payers, such as Medicare, will not accept such billing.

separate billing   Billing which clearly identifies hospital and physician services and charges (and thus permits their separation). This may be accomplished on a properly designed single bill, or through the use of two bills, one for the hospital and one for the physician.

blacklisting   Refusal by insurers to insure high-risk industries, professions, or individuals (especially those who might inherit diseases). If the blacklisting applies to high-risks in a given geographical area, it is called "redlining" (this has been a civil rights issue). Refusal to insure a high-risk industry is also called "industry screening."

Blue Cross (BC)   The nonprofit hospital care prepayment plan which was developed and sponsored by hospitals, and which originally was restricted to furnishing hospital care. Many BC plans have linked with their counterpart Blue Shield (BS) plans, which are physician sponsored, and which deal with physician (medical) care. Some 77 plans of each type, BC and BS, are in existence across the United States, and state statutes typically govern their operation. While plans are similar in principle, each one is autonomous; there are differences in policies, benefit structure, and administration from plan to plan. When the local BC and BS plans have linked, they are typically referred to jointly as Blue Cross/Blue Shield (BC/BS).

Blue Cross and Blue Shield (BC/BS)   The nonprofit health care prepayment plans (health insurance plans) which originated with hospitals and physicians, respectively. In many areas the Blue Cross (BC) and Blue Shield (BS) plans have merged. There are about 77 of these health insurance plans linked by a national association, the Blue Cross and Blue Shield Association (BCBSA).

Blue Cross and Blue Shield Association (BCBSA)   The national association of the nonprofit health care prepayment plans, originated by hospitals and physicians, respectively, called Blue Cross (BC) and Blue Shield (BS) plans. The original stimulus for the national association was to facilitate the BC and BS plans entering into "national" contracts, for example, with large corporations having plants or offices in the territories of several BC and BS plans, each of which has somewhat different policies and benefit structures.

Blue Indigo   The concept that (1) the health of a population is primarily its own responsibility and (2) health care reform, as well as achievement of improvement of individual health, can only be the result of the mobilization of local resources under community leadership. Innovation and experimentation are fundamental to the concept. The concept originated with a task force of the National Council of Community Hospitals (NCCH) and a parallel task force of the faculty of the Estes Park Institute (EPI). A national body, Indigo Institute, has been established to undertake further research, develop, and encourage the concept and to assist local communities in its adoption.

Blue Indigo Corporation   A corporation, typically a nonprofit (501(c)(3)) health-related corporation, which has been formed by a community in order to implement the Blue Indigo concept. As the concept develops, a few criteria must be met before a corporation can properly be called a Blue Indigo Corporation: (1) there must be collaborative effort between at least two local organizations, one of them a health care organization; but if there are only two organizations, only one of them should be a health care organization; (2) at least one of the organizations is *not* a governmental unit; (3) primary concern is *health* (rather than simply health *care*)—a Blue Indigo Corporation is not just a new kind of health care delivery system; (4) the organization must serve a defined population; (5) the corporation's efforts may be directed at the solution of any problem which affects the health of the local population, and which the corporation wants to address; (6) goals should be set in such a manner that it is possible to measure their achievement; such measurement is incumbent upon the corporation; (7) physicians and hospitals must participate, but the decision making is in the hands of a governing body which is representative of all the sponsors—i.e., health care providers only provide input along with the other partners in the Blue Indigo process, most importantly, community leaders; (8) only rarely would a state-wide organization qualify for the Blue Indigo Corporation label; the essence of the concept is that the community served be small enough to have common problems and interests.

Blue Shield (BS)   The nonprofit medical (physician) care prepayment plan which was developed by and sponsored by physicians, and which originally was restricted to furnishing physician care. Many BS plans have linked with their counterpart Blue Cross (BC) plans, which are hospital sponsored, and which deal with hospital care. Some 77 plans of each type, BC and BS, are in existence across the United States, and state statutes typically govern their operation. While plans are similar in principle, each one is autonomous; there are differences in policies, benefit structure, and administration among them from plan to plan. When the local BS and BC plans are linked, they are typically called jointly Blue Cross/Blue Shield (BC/BS).

board (governing)   A common term for the hospital's governing body, the body which is legally responsible for the hospital's policies, organization, management, and quality of care. "Board" is short for "board of trustees," "board of directors," or "board of governors." It is discussed further under *governing body*.

board of directors   See *governing body*.

board of trustees   See *governing body*.

boarder   A person, other than a patient, physician, or employee, who is temporarily residing in a hospital or other health care facility. A patient's parent or spouse staying in the hospital would be a boarder.

   boarder baby   pending.

bond   A certificate sold by a corporation or government entity to raise funds. It is basically a form of "IOU" upon which the corporation or government entity will pay interest to the bondholder for a given period of time, and pay the bondholder the amount borrowed (the principal amount) at the end of that time. Some bonds qualify as "tax-exempt," meaning that the bondholder does not have to pay taxes on the interest earned.

performance bond A bond which guarantees correct and timely performance (for example, construction of a facility) and which will pay money if the performance is not completed.

rapid amortization bond A bond with special provisions which permit the principal to be paid off without penalty (i.e., the bond may be retired) prior to its maturity date.

revenue bond A bond payable solely from the revenue generated from the operation of the project being financed, for which the bond was sold. In the case of hospital revenue bond financing, the bonds are typically payable from the gross receipts of the hospital. Such bonds may only be sold by municipalities (or by quasi-municipal organizations, such as hospitals, under special legislation).

tax-exempt bond A bond, the holder of which does not have to pay taxes on the interest she receives. Municipalities and, in some instances, nonprofit hospitals, are authorized to sell "tax-exempt" bonds.

bond indenture The contract between a bondholder and the institution (for example, a hospital) issuing the bond.

break-even analysis An analytical technique for studying the relation among fixed costs and variable costs (see *cost*), volume or level of activity (sales), and profits.

break-even chart A chart graphically presenting the results of a break-even analysis.

break-even point The volume of activity (for example, sales) where revenues and expenses are exactly equal, that is, the level of activity where there is neither a gain nor a loss from operations. Activity above the break-even point produces profits; activity below it results in losses.

browser A computer program used to read (browse) information on the Internet's World Wide Web.

budget neutrality A term which came into use as part of the prospective payment system (PPS) to mean that the new payment system may not pay hospitals, in the aggregate, any more or less for Medicare patients than the hospitals would have been paid under the previous system. More generally, a budget may be said to be "neutral" if, in total, it is neither larger than nor smaller than the previous budget.

budget reconciliation A part of the legislative budgeting process which defines federal programs in such a manner that program costs are consistent with Congress' decision as to how much money is to be spent for the program in question.

building codes Regulations which owners must meet in the construction, use, and maintenance of buildings. Building codes are promulgated and enforced by government agencies and are designed to ensure that buildings are durable and safe. The National Fire Protection Association (NHPA) issues, and periodically revises, a standard called the *Life Safety Code* which covers both construction and operation of buildings in such a manner as to maximize fire safety. While not strictly a building code, compliance with this code is required of hospitals wishing accreditation by the Joint Commission on Accreditation of Healthcare Organizations (JCAHO).

bundling Grouping things together into a package. See *global fee* and *unbundling*.

outpatient bundling A Health Care Financing Administration (HCFA) regulation which would require hospitals to "bundle" into the bill to Medicare diagnostic procedures or tests which are provided to a registered outpatient by outside suppliers, even though the service is provided outside the outpatient department. In the past, such services could be billed separately. The bundling would obtain for services that are the result of an outpatient "encounter," i.e., a direct personal contact between a patient and a physician or other person authorized to order services for patient diagnosis or treatment.

bylaws A document adopted by a corporation or association which governs its business conduct and the rights and responsibilities of its members. Bylaws may also authorize the separate issuance of rules and regulations to govern specific activities. The process for changing the rules and regulations is less cumbersome than that for changing the bylaws themselves.

hospital bylaws The bylaws of the hospital corporation, which cover such matters as how directors will be elected to the board of directors (governing body), their terms, how often they will meet, and so forth.

medical staff bylaws The portion of the bylaws of the hospital pertaining to the rights and obligations of physicians and others as members of the medical staff of the hospital. The medical staff bylaws cover medical staff governance, membership, privileges, discipline, and the like. Typically the bylaws are drafted and proposed by the medical staff, but they are approved and adopted by the hospital governing body, and their force stems from this governing body action. Serious consideration is being given to separating the traditional medical staff bylaws to retain organizational matters within the medical staff bylaws, but to create a separate policy on credentials matters (appointment, reappointment, and privileges) so that the separate documents may be more easily amended, if necessary, and to minimize potential legal problems (such as antitrust allegations, which may charge that the medical staff has too much control over credentials decisions if the process is entirely within the medical staff bylaws).

C

cafeteria plan Also referred to as a "flexible benefit plan", it allows participating employees to choose from a cafeteria-type menu of different health care coverage and provider options. If the cafeteria plan qualifies under Section 125 of the Internal Revenue Code (IRC), employees may also choose between non-taxable benefits and taxable cash. The advantages of one of these plans for employers is lower FICA

(Federal Insurance Contributions Act) and FUTA (Federal Unemployment Tax Act) taxes. The advantages for employees are being allowed to pick and choose benefits, and to pay for the benefits with before-tax dollars. See also *Zero Balanced Reimbursement Account (ZEBRA)*.

Canadian Council on Health Facilities Accreditation (CCHFA) The Canadian counterpart to the Joint Commission on Accreditation of Healthcare Organizations (JCAHO) in the United States. It was formerly called the Canadian Council on Hospital Accreditation (CCHA). Both CCHFA and JCAHO are voluntary bodies concerned with the quality of hospitals and other health care facilities. Originally JCAH (JCAHO's former name) performed its functions for hospitals in both the United States and Canada, but in 1955 CCHA was formed for Canadian hospitals.

Canadian Hospital Association (CHA) The national association of hospitals in Canada, the counterpart of the American Hospital Association (AHA) in the United States.

Canadian-style system This phrase is often used to describe a single-payer, nationalized or socialized health care system. Actually, Canada has a system consisting of national health insurance and twelve separate single-payer systems—the ten provinces plus two territories—each with a global budget (see *global budgeting*). Most physicians are self-employed and reimbursed under a negotiated fee schedule. Patients choose their own physicians. About half of the hospitals are government-owned; the rest are nonprofits which are reimbursed in lump sums. The provinces approve investments in facilities and technologies.

There are five key and indispensable principles of the Canadian system:
universality
comprehensiveness
accessibility
portability
public administration
Proponents of this plan contend that the absence of paperwork (compared with the U.S.) would save enough money to virtually eliminate the cost crisis, that physicians are free from interference in their decisions about patient care, that patients have freedom of choice, and that both physicians and patients like the system.

cap A limit on the amount of money which may be spent for a given purpose. A global budget for health care for a community would be such a cap.

out-of-pocket cap A maximum amount which an individual will be required to pay for health care in the form of copayments or deductibles in a given time period.

capital Usually, the long-term assets of the organization which are not bought and sold in the course of its operation. These assets are primarily fixed assets such as land, equipment, and building.

working capital The difference between current assets and current liabilities.

capital budgeting   The process of planning expenditures on capital items, that is, assets whose useful life is expected to extend beyond one year: property, plant, and equipment.

capital cost   See *capital cost* under *cost.*

capital expenditure   An expenditure (chargeable to an asset account) made to acquire an asset which has an estimated life in excess of one year and is not intended for sale in the ordinary course of business. It is also known as a capital expense. Expenses for operation (including maintenance) of the asset are not capital expenditures, but operating expenses.

capital expenditure review (CER)   See *capital expenditure review (CER)* under *review.*

capital financing   Obtaining funds for building or renovation, that is, for additions to capital, as opposed to the financing of operations. For the most part, operations are financed by fees for services rendered.

capital leverage   See *financial leverage* under *leverage.*

capital pass-through   Costs, such as depreciation and interest, which are "passed through." In other words, these costs are not included in the Diagnosis Related Group (DRG) prices, but are paid directly to the hospital in the prospective payment system (PPS).

capital rationing   A situation where a constraint is placed on the total size of capital investment during a particular period.

capital structure   The permanent long-term financing of an organization or institution represented by long-term debt, preferred stock, and net worth. Capital structure is distinguished from financial structure, which includes short-term debt plus all reserve accounts.

capitation   Capitation is a flat periodic payment to a physician or health care system per person cared-for ("per capita"). The provider assumes the risk that the payment will cover the costs for whatever the patient needs. Careful actuarial study beforehand in determining the amount of the fee makes this far less of a gamble than might be thought. Capitation has probably the lowest administrative cost of any payment mechanism.

   Capitation has been the most commonly mentioned form of payment in health care reform discussions, and an increasing number of managed care plans are employing this method of payment. Opponents allege that capitation offers too great a temptation to skimp on care in order to enhance profits. Proponents respond that avoiding this problem is one reason to emphasize quality measurements, and adequate supervision of the system.

captive insurance company   See *captive insurance company* under *insurance.*

care   The treatment and other services provided to a patient. Care is often described according to the needs of the patient: for example, neonatal care describes the care given newborns; respiratory care describes the care provided for patients with respiratory (breathing) difficulties. Care may also be described according to the "level" (intensity) or urgency of care, the health professional providing care, or the facility required. See also *level of care*.

Types of care, for example, include acute, adult day, after, ambulatory, basic nursing, bereavement, critical, custodial, day, elder, elective, emergency, home health, home life, hospice, hospital nursing, inpatient, intensive, intermediate, intermittent, life, long-term, managed, medical, personal, primary, progressive patient, rehabilitative, rehabilitative nursing, respite, rest home, secondary, self, skilled nursing, secondary, subacute, terminal, tertiary, transitional, uncompensated, and urgent.

caregiver   An individual who provides care for a disabled or ill friend or relative.

carrier (insurance)   An organization which handles the claims for beneficiaries on behalf of certain kinds of health insurance. A carrier may be an insurance company, a prepayment plan, or a government agency. In general, a carrier is at some risk. On the other hand, an intermediary, which is an agency in the Medicare system which has been selected to pay claims, and which is responsible only for taking care of the administration of the plan, is not at risk.

carrier (disease)   An individual who carries, and can transmit, a contagious disease without himself showing symptoms or signs of the disease.

carving out   A practice by insurers of providing group coverage only to healthy individuals in a small business, while permitting sicker co-workers to purchase only expensive high risk pool coverage. Carving out is a method of avoiding adverse selection. The practice is questionable and sometimes illegal.

case (health care)   A patient and his medical problem. Used alone, the term "patient" does not indicate whether the individual is ill or well. However, the term "case" denotes that the patient is ill, injured, or otherwise presents a problem to the health care provider. With a modifier or additional information, "case" describes the patient's problem, as, for example, a "case of influenza."

case (legal)   A controversy which is contested in a court of law. In common usage, a legal "case" refers to the particular facts of the controversy and the legal theories, allegations, and defenses being applied to those facts.

case management (patient care)   A traditional term for all the activities which a physician normally performs to insure the coordination of the medical services required by a patient. This is not the same function as that of the gatekeeper in managed care. Under ordinary circumstances, the American Medical Association (AMA) does not consider case management a separately reimbursable service.

case management (gatekeeping)   A term which, when used in connection with managed care, covers all the activities of evaluating the patient, planning treatment, referral, and follow-up, so that care is continuous and comprehensive and payment for the care is obtained. See *gatekeeper*.

case mix   The mix of cases, defined by age, sex, diagnoses, treatments, severity of illness, and so on, handled by a practitioner or hospital. Case mix is defined by: (1) grouping patients (classification) according to these factors; and then (2) determining the proportion of the total falling into each group. At present, the most widely used classification for this purpose is the Diagnosis Related Group (DRG) system. Sometimes the term "case mix" is used, inaccurately, to mean the grouping system itself (DRG, for example).

In the Medicare prospective payment system (PPS), which sets a price for each DRG, the total revenue for the hospital for its Medicare patients depends on how many "items" it "sells," and of what kind, that is, the number of patients cared for and the DRG of each. The revenue, therefore, is dependent upon the hospital's case mix.

case shifting   See *dumping.*

catastrophic illness   An illness which requires very costly treatment; one which is catastrophic to the patient's or family's finances. The illness may be either acute or chronic, and it may run its course quickly or over a protracted period.

catastrophic insurance   See *insurance.*

catchment area   See *service area.*

census   The number of patients in a hospital at a given time.

>   **average daily census (ADC)**   The average number of inpatients (see *patient*) in a hospital (or unit of the hospital, such as a patient care unit) each day for a given period of time. Newborns (born in the hospital) are not included in the inpatient count for calculation of this statistic.

>   **boarder census**   The number of boarders (non-patients residing temporarily) in a hospital.

center of excellence (COE)   A health care facility or department which has gained a reputation for superior quality in a special area (or areas) of care. Such a facility can bring in patients from great distances, and so can increase its expertise in its specialty while lowering the cost of care. A COE can also be used as a marketing tool to distinguish between providers.

Centers for Disease Control and Prevention (CDC)   A unit of the federal government (Department of Health and Human Services), with headquarters in Atlanta, Georgia, responsible for monitoring and study of diseases which are controllable by public health measures. New diseases which appear to occur in epidemics are investigated, as are those due to environmental problems. Here, for example, is the government's center for monitoring and research on acquired immunity deficiency syndrome (AIDS), toxic shock syndrome, and Legionnaire's disease.

>   CDC has four centers and one institute:
>   Center for Environmental Health
>   Center for Health Promotion and Education
>   Center for Infectious Diseases
>   Center for Prevention Services
>   National Institute for Occupational Safety and Health

certificate of need (CON)   A certificate, issued by a governmental or planning agency, which approves the hospital's contention that it needs a given facility or service (for example, open heart surgery). A certificate of need is required under many regulatory situations in order to obtain approval to build, purchase, or institute the service in question.

chain organization   See *multihospital system.*

channel system   A term sometimes given to a computer network system in which computer terminals in a number of locations are tied into a central location and information system. An example of a channel system is an airline network serving travel agents who can use their terminals in the system to do scheduling, determine fares, and sell tickets, with the central computer and information system handling all the transactions and creating the data displays.

Channel systems are being used in health care with the development of, for example, networks centered in a given hospital or health care system headquarters, with the remote terminals in physicians' offices, laboratories, and clinics. A number of tasks can be performed with this system. For example, a given physician's office can make appointments with other physicians and with hospitals. Such a system "channels" patients from the physicians who are in the network into other parts of the network rather than into other health care systems. The channel system is developed primarily to retain patients within the network, and to "feed" patients to the owner of the system, typically a hospital or other health care organization.

channeling   A term used in long-term care in which efforts are made to avoid institutionalization of patients by having them directed ("channeled") to community-based long-term care services. From 1980 to 1985, the Health Care Financing Administration (HCFA) and other federal agencies financed a demonstration of the concept, which used comprehensive case management, but ended the demonstration when a study showed no lowering of cost. More recently, reports suggest that when a *gatekeeper* participates in the financial planning as well as the health care decisions, significant savings may be realized.

charge   The dollar amount asked for a service by a health care provider. It is contrasted with the cost, which is the dollar amount the provider incurs in furnishing the service. It is difficult to determine precise costs for many services, and in such cases charges are substituted for costs in many reimbursement and payment formulas (often with the stipulation that the hospital's bookkeeping follow certain rules).

allowable charge   See *covered charge.*

covered charge   An item of service which, when billed to a third party payer, will be paid, since it is for a benefit provided under the contract. The charges for television and meals for visitors, for example, are not ordinarily covered charges. Synonym(s): allowable charge.

daily service charge   Same as "room rate"; see *room rate* under *rate (charge).*

charitable purpose Section 501(c)(3) of the Internal Revenue Code provides that one test of the qualification of an organization for tax-exemption under that Section of the code is that it serve a "charitable purpose." The term is defined adminsitratively by the Internal Revenue Service, and current regulations should be consulted.

charity allowance A reduction of a charge (a discount) to a patient because that patient is indigent or medically indigent.

cherry picking A practice by insurers of selling policies only to people who do not need medical care; then dropping them once they do. Any Medicare provider paid under a risk (capitated) plan, for instance, has an incentive to pursue this form of favorable selection. Some efforts to do this are illegal (such as asking Medicare HMO enrollees about their health status prior to joining), but it is apparently not illegal for HMO's to have their offices up one flight of stairs to discourage some potential enrollees, or to affirmatively market the HMO plan in environments frequented by the healthier retirees. Synonym(s): cream skimming.

chief executive officer (CEO) The person appointed by the governing body to direct the overall management of the hospital. The CEO is the "board in residence." Synonym(s): executive director.

chief financial officer (CFO) The corporate treasurer. Sometimes the term is also applied to the controller of the organization (the person in charge of the ongoing financial administration, including billing, accounting, budget management, and the like). Synonym(s): financial director.

chief information officer (CIO) The title often given to the person in charge of the organization's management information system (MIS) (see *information system*).

chief of nursing See *nursing service administrator*.

chief of service A medical staff officer responsible for the management of a clinical department, such as internal medicine or surgery. Synonym(s): chairman of service.

chief of staff The physician designated by the governing body, usually after nomination by the medical staff, to be responsible for management of the medical staff and for carrying out policy promulgated by the board. The term "chief of staff" or "president of the medical staff" usually refers to an unpaid person, while a paid physician with either of these same duties is likely to be called the "medical director," "vice president for medical affairs," "director of medical affairs" (DMA), or some like title.

There is some ambiguity in the duties and titles, because there really are two duties involved "at the top of the medical staff": (1) to provide management for the medical staff as a component of the hospital, and for this duty, the title "chief of staff" seems appropriate; and (2) to act as the "spokesperson" for the medical staff members, and for this duty, the title "president" seems more apt.

Many hospitals have two separate positions: a president (often unpaid), elected by the medical staff (and approved by the governing body) to represent the medical staff, and a director of medical affairs (or similar title), employed by the hospital, to manage medical staff affairs.

chief operating officer (COO)   The person in charge of the internal operation of the organization, for example, a hospital.   The chief executive officer (CEO), while responsible for the internal operation of the organization, also has external responsibilities with the governing body, with the community, with other institutions, and so on.   Often a single individual is made responsible for "inside" affairs, under the CEO.   This person would be the COO, whether or not he is given that title.

Child Abuse Amendments   Amendments, enacted in 1984, to the federal Child Abuse Prevention and Treatment Act concerning medical treatment decisions for seriously ill newborns.   The amendments added the term "withholding of medically indicated treatment" to the statutory definition of child neglect; this is now often referred to as "medical neglect."   The law was passed in response to the Baby Doe case, and makes it a form of neglect to fail to treat correctable, life-threatening conditions in a child unless in the physician's "reasonable medical judgment" (1) the child is irreversibly comatose, (2) treatment would be futile in saving the child's life, or (3) the treatment would be virtually futile and inhumane under the circumstances. States must require hospitals to report cases of suspected medical neglect to the child protective service agencies, and provide procedures for appropriate intervention. Synonym(s): Baby Doe Law.

CHIMIS   See *community health integrated management information system (CHIMIS)* under *information system.*

CHIPPA   See *community health planning agency.*

chiropractic   See *medicine.*

chronic   An illness which lasts for a long time, and usually without prospect of immediate change either for the better or the worse.   It is contrasted with acute, which refers to having a short course, which often is relatively severe.   "Chronic" is also used for the portion or portions of an illness, ordinarily in its later stages, in which symptoms are less severe and the patient may be at relatively low risk.

churning   The practice of discharge of a patient from the hospital and readmission of the same patient for what is really a single episode of care in order to be able to charge for two or more hospitalizations.   Only the last discharge is "real" from a medical standpoint—except for the financial benefit of being paid for two or more hospitalizations under the prospective payment system (PPS), there would have been no intermediate discharges.

price churning   See *predatory pricing.*

civil monetary penalty   A fine. "Civil" pertains to legal matters which are not criminal, but "penalty" means that the money to be paid is for punishment of the wrongdoer, rather than as compensation to the injured. Synonym: civil money penalty.

Civilian Health and Medical Program of the Uniformed Services (CHAMPUS)   A program that pays for medical care given by civilian providers to retired members of the uniformed services of the United States, and to the dependents of both active and retired members of these services. The program is administered by the Department of Defense.

Civilian Health and Medical Program of the Veterans Administration (CHAMPVA)
The federal program, administered by the Defense Department for the Veterans Administration, which provides care for the dependents of totally-disabled veterans. Care is given by civilian providers.

claim (insurance)   A request for payment of insurance benefits to be paid to or on behalf of a beneficiary.

claim (legal)   An allegation of legal liability and an accompanying demand for damages (money) or other rights due. The term is sometimes used in health care to refer to a medical malpractice lawsuit, or to an allegation of malpractice (which allegation may or may not result in a lawsuit).

claims filing service   A service offered by private entrepreneurs to Medicare beneficiaries and others with health insurance. The service offers to "file, follow-up, and manage" claims (see *claim*). Often the service charges a "registration" fee plus monthly fees. Such a service, which costs perhaps $100 per beneficiary per year, adds to the cost of health care by that amount and, equally importantly, decreases the individual's benefits by that amount.

claims-made coverage   See *claims-made coverage* under *insurance coverage*.

claims processing   The procedure by which claims for payment for services are reviewed in order to determine whether they should be paid, and for what amount (see *claim*). The review includes verifying that an authorized provider is submitting the claim, that the person served is a beneficiary, that the services are medically reasonable and are for available benefits, and the amount to be paid.

claims review   See *claims review* under *review*.

Clayton Act   One of the primary federal antitrust laws. The Clayton Act specifically prohibits price discrimination (selling to different buyers at different, discriminatory prices) (Section 2(a), as amended by the Robinson-Patman Act), tying arrangements, exclusive dealing, and corporate expansion if these activities substantially lessen competition or create a monopoly. It also prohibits interlocking corporate directorships where the corporations are competitors; no individual may simultaneously serve on the boards of directors of two or more competing corporations, if one of the corporations has assets over one million dollars. 15 U.S.C. secs. 12 *et seq.* (1982).

client   A person who receives professional services. In health care, a client may or may not be sick.

clinic (facility)   A facility for ambulatory patients.

free clinic   Exactly what the name implies: a volunteer facility which provides free care, primarily to the working poor. About 200 such clinics are in operation in the United States, the first of this generation being the Haight-Ashbury Free Clinic which was established in San Francisco in 1967. Free clinics usually offer medical care in the form of physical examinations, prenatal care, family planning, and primary care for their clientele. Some may also provide dental health care and mental health services, while others offer social and legal services. Financing is usually by donations. A great deal of the staff are volunteers. Supplies are often provided at a discount, and space may be donated, e.g., by churches.

clinic (education) An instructional session, such as a prenatal clinic where expectant mothers are instructed in their own care and prepared for the care of their babies. In medical education, a clinic is where students are taught by demonstration with actual patients.

clinic (practice) A group of physicians practicing together, either all of one specialty (single specialty) or with various specialties (multispecialty). Such a clinic may or may not have inpatient facilities.

clinical A term referring to direct contact with or information from patients and to the course of illness; "things" medical about a patient. Thus personal (bedside) contact with the patient is clinical contact, a laboratory which examines blood and other specimens from patients is a clinical laboratory, the patient's medical record is a clinical record, research involving patients is clinical research, a nurse taking care of patients is a clinical nurse.

clinical care path See *critical path*.

Clinical Information System (CLICKS) See *Clinical Information System (CLICKS)* under *information system*.

clinical privileges See *privileges*.

clinical record See *medical record*.

code creep See *DRG creep*.

coded Hospital jargon referring to a patient for whom a code blue signal has been sent, indicating the occurrence of a cardiac (heart) emergency. Similarly, when a do not resuscitate order (DNR) has been recorded for a patient, that patient, in hospital jargon, is "not to be coded" (resuscitated).

cognitive services A term applied to all the activities of a physician (or other professional) other than the performance of procedures. The charges of physicians are relatively easy to explain in surgery and other instances where "something is done" to the patient. High charges for, say, diagnostic evaluations, patient and family counseling, and the care of patients with infectious diseases, are much harder to explain, and thus charges are considerably lower. "Cognitive services" require as much time and skill as surgery. However, much of this effort and skill is simply not seen by the patient or payer. Nonetheless, an education as long and arduous as the surgeon's may be required, as well as unseen time in the library and informal consultation with colleagues. Efforts to overcome the resulting perceived inequities in payment have led to the labeling of non-procedural services as cognitive (intellectual). No term for "non-cognitive" services seems to have appeared.

coinsurance A percentage to be paid by a health care plan enrollee (beneficiary) of the cost of health care services. For example, the enrollee have a 50% coinsurance contract, which requires the enrollee to pay 50% of the charge amount which has been approved for that service by the plan. The health plan pays its portion of the charge (50% in this case) and sends the enrollee an Explanation of Benefits which shows the amount owed by the enrollee. The enrollee sends payment directly to the provider of the service. This is a method of cost-sharing between the enrollee and the plan, and serves as an incentive for the enrollee to stay healthy and to use heatlh care resources wisely, thus helping to contain health care costs. See also *copayment* and *deductible*.

collateral source rule   A legal rule of evidence which prohibits the jury from considering the fact that the plaintiff has been compensated from any source other than the defendant. The practical result is that a medical malpractice defendant may have to pay the full amount of the plaintiff patient's medical and other expenses, even if the patient has already received reimbursement for those expenses from another source, such as medical insurance.

collegial   The sharing of power or authority equally among a number of colleagues. In a truly collegial environment, no one individual can be held accountable since no one individual is in charge.

comfort care   Medical or other health care whose sole or primary purpose is the comfort of the patient. In the Oregon plan, comfort care is defined to include health services which are diagnostic, curative, or focused on active treatment of the primary condition and intended to prolong life. Examples of comfort care include pain medication, hospice services, medical equipment and supplies (beds, wheelchairs, etc.), palliative services for symptom relief (e.g. radiation therapy).

Commission on Professional and Hospital Activities (CPHA)   An independent non-profit organization based in Ann Arbor, Michigan, dedicated to the improvement of health care quality through the use of comparative data. It was formed in 1955 with the national sponsorship of the American College of Physicians (ACP), the American College of Surgeons (ACS), and the American Hospital Association (AHA). CPHA provides certain shared clinical and management information services (MIS) data processing, performs interpretive research services for hospitals and other health care institutions, and disseminates information to the health care field. Its largest and oldest program is the prototype hospital discharge abstract system, the Professional Activity Study (PAS).

Communitarian Network   A Washington DC-based group which advocates shared responsibility and community-based decision making. A recent paper, "Core Values in Health Care Reform," proposes that it is important that health care reforms not undermine the culture of care in their pursuit of savings and improvement of access.

Community Care Network™ (CCN)   This term has been adopted as the service mark for Community Care Networks, Inc. and San Diego Community Healthcare Alliance, which reserve all rights to its use. The term is also used (with the service mark indicated) by the American Hospital Association for the kind of community health care organization which it promotes. The service mark must be employed because of its reservation by the California organizations. The network would consist of local groups of physicians and clinics, organized by hospitals, competing for contracts with group insurers to provide care to enrolled individuals. The payment schedule would be established by an independent regulatory board, and providers would normally be reimbursed on a capitated basis.

community care plan (CCP)   The Eutaw Group's alternative to (or complement to) the accountable health plan (AHP) in the health care reform movement (1993). A CCP is expected to carry out a proactive "predict and manage" philosophy; its proponents see the AHP as essentially a "treat and/or prevent what comes in the door" organization. It is directed at "equal health status" rather than "equity in prices per capita," as it describes the AHP's goal. A CCP would offer (1) "essential gateway services," accessible via a "gatekeeper mechanism " in the hands of a generalist (physician or allied health professional, with physician oversight; see *gatekeeper* and (2) "essential referral services."

The gatekeeper services would consist of "assessment of health needs via surveillance, outreach, and screening, using traditional public health approaches and nontraditional proactive health (home and school) visitors; entry to care networks; child and adult therapeutic and preventive generalist care; emergency services; AIDS counseling; sexually transmitted disease (STD) intervention; family planning; maternity care; nutrition services; mental health services; dental services; social support; transportation; and home health." The referral services would include hospital care ranging from full service down to "essential access" community hospitals, hospice, nursing home, and rehabilitation. The West Alabama Health Services project in Eutaw County, Alabama, is a prototype program of the Eutaw Group.

Community Health Accreditation Program (CHAP)   A program of a subsidiary of the National League for Nursing (NLN) for evaluating and elevating the quality of home health care programs, their management, and their outcomes. Those programs meeting the standards of CHAP are given accreditation. The standards pertain to planning, finance, service delivery, operations, human resources, evaluation, and outcomes of care.

community health center (CHC)   A term used loosely to cover community, migrant, and homeless health centers. Over 30 years ago, the federal government established a network of community and migrant health centers through grants from the U.S. Public Health Service. There are now 571 of these centers. Two-thirds of their patients are women and children. The centers employ or contract for the services of 3,600 physicians as well as other providers. To these centers have been added 119 homeless health centers through the Health Care for the Homeless Programs, also with funds from the U.S. Public Health Service. The total is 690 centers. All together, they provide comprehensive preventive and primary health services to medically underserved populations, both rural and urban, of more than 7,000,000 people at 1,400 sites across the country, including Puerto Rico and the District of Columbia. The centers are built on a public-private partnership and are supported by federal, state, and local funds, as well as by private sources. The term includes "neighborhood health centers," "family health centers," and "community health networks (CHNs)." Sometimes called a "Section 330" [of the Public Health Service Act] health services group. [Further information can be obtained from the National Association of Community Health Centers, Inc.]

community health integrated management information system (CHIMIS)   See *community health integrated management information system (CHIMIS)* under *information system.*

Community Health Intervention Partnerships (CHIPs)   Projects of the Hospital Research and Educational Trust (HRET) of the American Hospital Association (AHA) under a grant from the Robert Wood Johnson Foundation designed to help hospitals and health systems work with community development corporations to assess local health needs, identify major community health problems, and develop plans to address them (1995).

community health network (CHN)   A term sometimes employed as a label for a municipally operated system of providing health care for the poor.

community health planning agency (CHIPPA)   The term employed in Florida for the organizations established by statute in 1993 to serve the same function as health alliances (HAs). The state is to be covered by 11 of these agencies.

community health services   A term which encompasses preventive procedures, diagnosis, and treatment for residents of a community. It does not imply any organizational structure.

community health worker (CHW)   A community member who serves as a connector between health care providers and health care consumers. Most of the work is done in the community setting among groups which have traditionally been underserved.   The CHW identifies community health problems, develops innovative solutions, and translates the solutions into practice. Sometimes called a "lay health provider".

Community Medical Network Society (COMNET Society) ‘ A nonprofit membership organization founded in 1994 to bring together industries interested in community health *information* management. Members include providers, purchasers, payors, and physician groups along with vendors and consultants.

community rating   See *community rating* under *rating.*

community resource management (CRM)   The concept, in health care, that the unit which should be considered in the allocation of resources is the entire community rather than each of its component organizations.

comorbidity   See *comorbidity* under *morbidity.*

compensable   Something for which the law allows money to be awarded to make amends or restore someone to their prior position.   Not all types of injury (for example, mental distress suffered by an unusually sensitive person) are compensable. See *damages.*
  In workers' compensation law, "compensable" describes an injury or illness which is work-related, and therefore covered by the workers' compensation system.

compensation   In addition to the common meaning of payment for work done, compensation covers systems to make reparation for damage or injury done. Traditionally, patients who have been injured by the health care system, either by malpractice or otherwise, have sought compensation by filing a claim—which usually results in a lawsuit—against the health care provider. This system is lengthy and costly, and does not always provide a fair result. Thus, alternatives are being proposed.

neo-no-fault compensation See *patients' compensation.*

no-fault compensation A system of compensation for persons who have been injured or adversely affected, without the need to prove fault or wrongdoing. No-fault systems are presently in use to compensate auto and industrial accident victims (see *workers' compensation*). Several no-fault (or no-fault-like) plans have been suggested for the health care area; see, for example, *patients' compensation.*

patients' compensation A no-fault system for compensating patients who suffer harm as a result of some aspect of medical or hospital care, proposed as an alternative to malpractice litigation. Synonym(s): neo-no-fault compensation.

workers' compensation (WC) A system of compensating workers for on-the-job injuries, developed as an alternative to lawsuits by injured employees. The typical workers' compensation law compensates workers who suffer work-related injuries (regardless of fault), and provides that workers' compensation benefits are the "exclusive remedy," the only means of receiving compensation for work-related injuries and illnesses. Workers may therefore not sue their employers. Workers' compensation was formerly called workmen's compensation.

compensation fund See *alternative dispute resolution (ADR).*

competitive medical plan (CMP) A health care plan, licensed by the state, which provides health care services to enrolled members on a prepaid, capitated basis. Most often used to refer to an entity (can be an HMO as well as a competitive medical plan) which has met certain requirements of the federal government to be designated as a competitive medical plan. A federally designated CMP is eligible for a risk contract with HCFA to provide Medicare services to Medicare beneficiaries. The requirements for CMP designation are not as strict as those for becoming federally qualified.

comprehensive health care Services that are intended to meet all the health care needs of a patient: outpatient, inpatient, home care, and other.

comprehensive health care delivery system A health care delivery system which includes both facilities and professionals, and which is set up to provide comprehensive health care to a defined population.

comprehensive health planning (CHP) See *planning.*

comprehensive health planning agency (CHP agency) An agency established in response to a federal health planning act in 1966, which was later replaced by a group of agencies established under federal legislation passed in 1974. The latter agencies were the health systems agencies (HSAs), state health planning and development agencies, and statewide health coordinating councils (SHCCs).

compression of morbidity See *compression of morbidity* under *morbidity.*

comptroller   See *controller.*

computer   A machine, typically electronic, that is capable of performing computations on data that is fed into it. The computations performed are governed by instructions given to the computer. The physical machinery itself is generally referred to as hardware, while the instructions given to the computer are referred to as software, or programs.

Since the widespread appearance of microprocessor chips in the 1980's, a variety of medical devices now contain computers to increase their capabilities. Not just limited to the common notion of a big box with a keyboard and TV-type screen attached to it, computers now control consumer electronics, cars, power tools, and washing machines.

mainframe computer   A computer with one or more central processing units (CPUs) designed to be used by many "users" at one time, and usually run by one or more "operators." Its processing and output facilities are accessed via computer terminals, and it is usually kept physically separate from users, typically in a climate controlled environment with restricted access and a sophisticated fire extinguishing system. A mainframe is distinguished from its smaller counterparts, the "mini" and "micro" (personal) computers, although the distinctions are becoming increasingly blurry.

microcomputer   A computer distinguishable from a minicomputer and a mainframe computer in that its "brain," the central processing unit (CPU), is a microprocessor chip. Microcomputers typically contain CPUs manufactured by Intel or Motorola, who have given these chips cryptic names such as 8088, 80386SX, or 68000, although by the mid-1990's names like Pentium and PowerPC were replacing numbers. The lines distinguishing micro, mini, and mainframe computers continue to get blurrier, as today's small computers outperform yesterday's large computers. Synonym(s): PC, personal computer.

neurocomputer   A computer or computer program which performs in a similar manner to the network of nerve cells in the brain. Other computers work by taking steps serially, that is, one step after another. However, in a neurocomputer, a number of elements of the computer work simultaneously. A neurocomputer can "learn," it can program itself, and it is especially good at pattern recognition. Synonym(s): neural computer, neural network machine, artificial neural system, electronic neural network, parallel associative network, parallel distributed processor, sixth generation computer.

sixth generation computer   See *neurocomputer.*

computer-based patient record (CPR)   See *computer-based patient record (CPR)* under *medical record.*

Computer-Based Patient Record Institute (CPRI)   An organization formed in 1991 to establish routine use of a computer-based patient record (CPR) system in all health care settings. Its formation was recommended in a study by the Institute of Medicine (IOM), The *Computer-Based Patient Record*, which was published earlier in 1991. The study called for fully-automated medical records in hospitals by the end of the decade. Advocates contend that such a record would radically change health care delivery by improving efficiency, quality of care, and cost containment. CPRI was formed by a coalition of about 35 interested groups, which included the American Medical Association (AMA), the American Health Information Management Association (AHIMA), and the US Chamber of Commerce. Membership is for corporations only (there were in 1995 approximately fifty corporate members); there are no individual memberships, although individuals may obtain the newsletter and participate in certain activities and work groups. Additional and updated information is available on CPRI's Internet web home page at http://www.CPRI.org.

computer decision support system (CDSS) See *decision support software (DSS)*.

computer hardware See *hardware*.

computer modeling The use of computers to design and test real world structures and processes, relying on the computers' ability to process vast amounts of data and perform complex mathematical calculations. In AIDS research, for instance, computer modeling could be used to study the effect of the virus on a variety of genetic structures which might be impossible to produce in the laboratory.

computer terminal A mechanical device used by persons to communicate with a computer. It typically has a keyboard and cathode ray tube (CRT) display. The terminal may be directly connected ("hardwired") to the "host" computer, or may use telephone lines via a modem. Increasingly, personal computers (PCs) are being used as terminals in addition to their other uses.

Computerized Patient Information System (CPIS) See *information system*.

concurrent review See *concurrent review* under *review*.

conflict of interest A situation where a person (or organization) has two separate and distinct duties owed concerning, or interests in, the same thing, and therefore cannot act completely impartially with respect to that thing. It is like one servant trying to serve two masters. For example, a hospital trustee has a legal duty to act in the best interests of the hospital. If that trustee owns real estate that the hospital wishes to buy, the trustee has a personal interest in obtaining the highest price, but as a trustee he has an interest in obtaining the lowest price. Since such a conflict of interest may cloud his judgment, the trustee is obligated to inform the hospital board about his personal interest, and usually will excuse himself from participating in the purchase negotiations. Even if there is no real conflict, or if the trustee is capable of making the right decision for the hospital, he would be wise to excuse himself so that the transaction will not appear to be tainted with impropriety, and so that no one can challenge it as such. Most corporate bylaws address conflict of interest situations.

Congressional Budget Office (CBO) An organization, created by the Congressional Budget Act of 1974, which provides the U.S. Congress with analyses of alternative fiscal, programmatic, and budgetary issues. It has been involved in studying and making recommendations concerning the costs of alternative health care reform proposals.

consent, informed   A legal term referring to the patient's right to make his own treatment decisions, based upon knowledge of the relevant alternatives and the benefits and risks of each. An "informed consent" is the consent of the patient after he has been fully informed, by the physician proposing the treatment or procedure, of the risks, benefits, and alternatives. Failure to obtain informed consent prior to surgery or administration of treatment may result in legal liability. An exception is ordinarily made in case of an emergency where the patient is unable to consent (e.g. he is unconscious), in which case the law presumes that the patient would have consented to the emergency treatment required to protect his life or health.

Although it is wise for the physician and hospital to obtain the written consent of the patient prior to a treatment or procedure, the patient's signature should not be confused with the consent itself. That is, the piece of paper is evidence of the patient's consent, but the essence of the informed consent is the patient's voluntary agreement based upon the relevant facts which have been communicated to the patient by the physician. Thus, a patient groggy from anesthesia who is asked to "sign this" on the way into the operating suite has not given informed consent.

Special conditions apply in biomedical research and with respect to comatose patients (subjects). Here a limited class of exempt research has been defined; waivers are allowed under certain conditions, and the concepts of "deferred consent" and "minimal differential risk" have been developed.

Consolidated Omnibus Budget Reconciliation Act of 1985 (COBRA)   A federal law which requires (among other things) that employers of 20 or more workers must continue former employees' health insurance coverage (at the former employee's expense) for up to three years for qualified beneficiaries. Qualified beneficiaries include widows and divorced and separated spouses of former employees, as well as their dependents (even dependents who lost their dependent status). The law amends the Internal Revenue Code of 1954.

consolidation   The formal union of two or more corporations (such as hospitals) into a single corporation. In a consolidation, all of the corporations which unite cease to exist, and a new corporation is formed with its own new identity. A merger is similar to a consolidation, except that one of the original corporations retains its identity and continues to exist, while the other corporations are merged into it and lose their former identities. In either case, the surviving or consolidated corporation acquires the assets and assumes the liabilities of the former corporations.

consortium   An alliance between two or more parties (for example, hospitals) to achieve a specific purpose.

consultation (medical)   A review of a patient's problem by a second individual, namely a physician or other health care provider (for example, a clinical psychologist), and the rendering of an opinion and advice to the referring physician. The review in most instances involves the independent examination of the patient by the consultant. In a consultation some evidence, such as X-rays, may not need to be repeated if it is made available to the consultant. The consultant's opinion and advice are not binding on the referring physician. A "second opinion" is a special kind of consultation in which a second surgeon consults on the desirability of elective surgery which has been recommended by the first surgeon. (Elective surgery is surgery which is not stated to be necessary to preserve life or prevent serious disability.)

consultation (management)   Advice from an expert, given after a study of a situation or problem presented by the individual obtaining the consultation. In the health care field, such consultation often concerns organization, management, strategic planning, personnel policies, and the like.

consumer   An individual who does or may receive health care services. In the context of health care programs or legislation, a consumer is not a provider. See also *customer*.

consumer choice   A reform approach which would get individuals to purchase health insurance by making it mandatory but providing a tax break; the poor would get a tax refund. Companies providing insurance would not get a tax break. Also called the "market-based approach."

consumer health informatics   Making health information directly available to consumers by electronic methods. Includes data banks ready to be installed on one's own computer, such as reference material from the Mayo Clinic; computer networks; use of voice mail systems — any electronic method.

consumer price index (CPI)   See *consumer price index (CPI)* under *index*.

contingency fee   A fee which is paid to an attorney only if the client wins. Contingency-fee arrangements are commonly used in malpractice cases, where the attorney receives a portion (usually about one-third) of the amount awarded the plaintiff by the court or in an out-of-court settlement. If the plaintiff receives nothing, the attorney receives nothing (except reimbursement of expenses).

contingent worker   A person who works less than 35 hours a week (or in some usages, less than 12 months a year). Such individuals typically have lower earnings, less job security, and fewer promotions than full-time employees. Contingent workers are often without health insurance. Synonym(s): peripheral workers, marginal workers.

continued stay review   See *continued stay review* under *review*.

continuing care retirement community (CCRC)   A retirement community which offers lifetime independent living and various health care services to residents.

continuity of care   The degree to which the care of a patient from the onset of illness until its completion is continuous, that is, without interruption. Interruptions occur sometimes because the patient does not follow through, sometimes because the system has gaps, often because of lack of facilities or because of financial impediments (absence of benefits, for example, which cover certain services). The term "continuity of care" is sometimes used to refer to a longer span of time than the single episode of illness, and to the patient's health care when he is both well and ill.

continuous quality improvement (CQI)   See *continuous quality improvement (CQI)* under *quality improvement*.

contract   An agreement between two or more parties which gives legally enforceable rights and obligations to both. A contract need not be in writing to be enforceable, unless it is a certain kind of agreement, such as one for the sale of real estate. A state law called the "Statute of Frauds" specifies which contracts must be supported by written evidence.

cost-plus contract   A type of agreement, often used in construction, in which the owner agrees to pay for all costs incurred by the contractor in executing the plans and specifications, "plus" an additional amount (fixed sum, percentage, or other arrangement) as a fee or profit.

exclusive contract   A term which, in the hospital, usually refers to a written agreement under which a given physician or physician group is given the exclusive right to furnish certain, specified administrative or clinical services in the hospital. During the life of the exclusive contract, other physicians are precluded from the same activities in that hospital. Exclusive contracts have raised antitrust issues for hospitals; see *Rule of Reason*.

indemnity contract   A health care insurance contract in which the benefits are money (cash) rather than service.

risk contract   A contract under which a provider agrees to furnish a given service for a prearranged fee, and thus assumes the risk (financial) that the fee will cover its costs for providing the service. A health maintenance organization (HMO) which operates under a capitation method of payment is a risk contractor.

service contract   A health care insurance contract in which the benefits are the actual services rather than money.

contract management   See *contract management* under *management*.

contract provider organization (CPO)   See *preferred provider organization*.

contract service   A service purchased from a person or another organization. If a hospital does not operate its own laundry or laboratory, for example, these may be obtained as contract services. Similarly, the physician services for an emergency department may be obtained by contract with an organization set up to furnish such services.

contractual adjustment   See *contractual adjustment* under *adjustment*.

control   The term used by the American Hospital Association (AHA) in its listing of hospitals in the Guide to the Health Care Field (AHA Guide) to indicate the kind of organization or institution responsible for operating the hospital. Some 24 categories are used. In the non-federal sector, the grouping is quite general, such as "church-operated" and "investor-owned (for-profit), partnership." In the federal sector, however, classification is much more specific; for example "Army" hospitals are separated from "Navy" hospitals.

controller The person who is in charge of the hospital's ongoing financial administration, including billing, accounting, budget management, and the like. A controller may or may not be the chief financial officer (CFO) (treasurer). "Controller" is sometimes spelled "comptroller."

conversion Retaining health insurance when changing employers without having to be reevaluated as to insurability. An employee retiring or otherwise ineligible to remain in a group usually converts to an individual health insurance policy. The privilege to convert in this manner is guaranteed in many circumstances by the Consolidated Omnibus Budget Reconciliation Act of 1985 (COBRA).

conversion factor A dollar amount for one base unit in the relative value scale (RVS). The price to be paid to the provider for a given service equals the relative value of the service multiplied by the dollar amount of the conversion factor. For example, a blood sugar determination might have a relative value of 5.0, and the conversion factor might be $5.00. The "price" of the blood sugar determination would therefore be $25.00.

cooperative care Care provided by family and friends, as in earlier times. These caregivers must work together cooperatively to ensure that the needs of the patient are met at all times. For example, family members may reside with the patient and handle much of the care; friends and neighbors may take turns giving needed therapies and providing relief for the primary caregivers. Cost savings of 30-40% in labor and similar savings in capital, as well as shorter institutional stays, are reported for patients who receive cooperative care (when appropriate). Fewer falls and fewer medication errors, as well as greater patient satisfaction, have been reported compared with traditional inpatient care. Cooperative care can be appropriate for both acute bedfast and ambulatory inpatients, with such conditions as hysterectomy, laparoscopy, arthroscopy, cosmetic surgery, and medical problems. Home bound patients may also receive such care, such as those with chronic or terminal conditions.

cooperative services See *shared services* under *service*.

coordination of benefits (COB) An insurance claims review process used when a beneficiary is insured by two or more carriers (see *claim*). The process determines the liability of each carrier in order to eliminate duplication of payments. For example, benefits to which an individual is entitled under workers' compensation are not permitted to be duplicated by ordinary health insurance, even though the injury or illness would be covered were the problem not work-related.

copayment A fixed amount of money paid by a health care plan enrollee (beneficiary) at the time of service. For example, the enrollee may pay a $10 "copay" at every physician office visit, and $5 for each drug prescription filled. The health plan pays the remainder of the charge directly to the provider. This is a method of cost-sharing between the enrollee and the plan, and serves as an incentive for the enrollee to use heatlh care resources wisely. An enrollee might be offered a lower price benefit package in return for a higher copayment. See also *coinsurance* and *deductible*.

core service(s)   Those services which must be provided by an institution if it is to be accepted by the American Hospital Association (AHA) as an institution eligible for registration with AHA and inclusion in the annual Guide to the Health Care Field (AHA Guide). These services include an organized medical staff, a nursing service with registered nurse (RN) supervision, food service, pharmacy, and maintenance of medical records.

corporate liability   See *corporate liability* under *liability*.

corporation   A legal entity which exists separately, for all legal purposes, from the people or organizations which own it. To take advantage of legal advantages (limitation of liability and tax benefits, for example), a corporation must observe certain "formalities" required by law, such as meetings, minutes, and filing of annual reports and tax returns.

for-profit corporation   A corporation whose profits (excess of income over expenses) are distributed, as dividends, to shareholders who own the corporation (in contrast to a nonprofit corporation, in which the profits go to corporate purposes rather than to individual shareholders).

medical staff corporation   Sometimes a medical staff incorporates itself, and the matters which are ordinarily the subject of the medical staff bylaws are then handled by contract between the medical staff corporation and the hospital corporation, much as an emergency services corporation could be contracted with to provide emergency department services.

nonprofit corporation   A corporation whose profits (excess of income over expenses) are used for corporate purposes rather than returned to shareholders or investors (owners) as dividends. To qualify for tax exemption, no portion of the profits of the corporation may "inure" to the benefit of an individual. See *inurement*. "Nonprofit" does not necessarily mean "tax-exempt". See also *501(c)(3)*.

parent corporation   A corporation which owns at least a majority of the shares of (controls) one or more subsidiary corporations.

professional corporation (PC)   A corporation in which all of the shareholders (owners) are members of a given profession, such as physicians. In some respects, a professional corporation is not the same as other corporations. One difference is that persons who are not members of the profession forming the corporation may not be shareholders (for example, physicians may not be shareholders of a legal PC). Another difference is that unlike a normal business corporation, the liability of a PC is not limited; in other words, its owners can be held personally liable for the PC's debts. A PC may also be called a "professional service corporation," "professional association," or "service corporation."

service corporation (SC)   See *professional corporation*.

subsidiary corporation   A corporation of which another corporation (the "parent corporation") owns at least a majority of the shares.

cost   The expense incurred in *providing* a product or service.

allowable cost   Items of service which are contractually included in the benefits of an insurance or payment plan, similar to "covered charges" (see *charge*). The charges for television and meals for visitors are not ordinarily allowable costs.

capital cost   The cost of developing or acquiring new equipment, facilities, or services; that is, the investment cost to the institution of such growth.

direct cost   A cost which can be identified directly with any part of the hospital organization which the hospital designates as a cost center. In fact, cost centers are defined as such because they are segments of the hospital, such as the operating rooms, to which direct costs can be assigned rather clearly. To the direct costs of each cost center are added, on the basis of some accounting formula, allocated proportions of the hospital's indirect costs (costs, such as for heat and housekeeping, which are not easily allocated to specific cost centers).

fixed cost   A cost which is entirely independent of the volume of activity. If no charges are made for individual local calls, the cost of local telephone service is a fixed cost; on the other hand, long distance service, which depends as it does on the number and length of calls made, is a variable cost (however, an unlimited WATS line would be a fixed cost).

indirect cost   There are two kinds of indirect costs in a hospital. The first kind is costs which must be incurred by any organization furnishing services, but which cannot be exactly identified with any specific service rendered or support department. For example, the cost of having a chief executive officer (CEO) is necessary, but it cannot be charged directly to, for example, the operating room as can the salaries of operating room nurses. The second kind of indirect costs is the costs of "support activities," the costs of which can be determined, but which do not produce revenue. Such activities (for example, a hospital's medical record department) have clear direct costs, and must bear their share of the indirect costs of the first type above. But, since these activities do not produce revenue, their costs—both direct and indirect—become indirect costs for the revenue-producing departments and services.   Accountants have developed a variety of formulas for "cost allocation." Cost allocation means assigning appropriate portions of the indirect costs to the various cost centers and then further allocating the costs of non-revenue-producing cost centers to the revenue-producing cost centers, where they influence the charges.

marginal cost   The addition to total cost resulting from the production of an additional unit of service or product. This cost varies with the volume of the operation. A hospital, for example, has a high cost for its first meal served. Subsequent meals have much lower costs each (marginal costs) until the volume is so large as to require changes in facilities, supervision, and the like. At this point the marginal cost will usually rise until a new equilibrium ("optimum output level") is established.

pass-through cost   A term with a specific definition in the prospective payment system (PPS). It refers to hospital costs, such as for medical education, which are not incorporated in the Diagnosis Related Group (DRG) prices. Funds are provided to the hospital directly, that is, outside the per-case payments for patient care; the costs are simply passed through (or outside of) the DRG mechanism.

reasonable cost   A term with a specific definition given by the federal government for use in Medicare. It is used only in connection with services in institutions which are exempt from the prospective payment system (PPS) and for beneficiaries who are not inpatients.

semi-variable cost   A cost which is partly a variable cost and partly a fixed cost in its behavior in response to changes in volume. Automobile rental is typically a semi-variable cost, with a fixed charge per day and a variable charge depending on miles driven.

variable cost   A cost which is entirely dependent on the volume of activity, as opposed to a fixed cost, which is not affected by volume. In a typical telephone billing system, for example, long distance calls represent a variable cost while local calls represent a fixed cost.

cost allocation   An accounting procedure by which costs that cannot be clearly identified with any specific cost center are distributed among cost centers, and by which the costs of support services are distributed among revenue-producing services so as to be recovered in the charges.

cost-benefit analysis   A technique for placing a numerical value on the benefits to be derived from using a piece of equipment or operating a program as compared with its costs. The goal is to develop a cost-benefit ratio. If the ratio is greater than 1.0, the benefits more than outweigh the costs; if the ratio is less than 1.0, the costs are greater than the benefits. This process is difficult to use in health care in many instances where the benefits are in quality of life rather than something readily measured in dollars.

cost-benefit ratio   See *cost-benefit ratio* under *ratio*.

cost center   An area of activity of the hospital with which direct costs can be identified. Accounting practice is to assign direct costs to such cost centers, and to allocate to each cost center its proportionate share of indirect costs, in order to give management a tool for cost control (or pricing). When a cost center is also revenue-producing, that is, an area for which charges are made (for example, an operating room), the allocation of direct and indirect costs, along with data about the services rendered, permits the charge for each service to be sufficient to cover the cost of that service.

Some other cost centers, over which management wants to maintain control, do not produce revenue. An example is the medical record department. The costs of such departments (direct plus indirect costs) are reallocated as indirect costs to the revenue-producing cost centers.

cost containment   Efforts to prevent increase in cost or to restrict its rate of increase. Cost containment is rarely addressed at reducing cost.

cost control   A term usually applied to an external constraint of costs (or charges), such as legislation or the actions of a regulatory agency.

cost-effective   Providing a service at a "reasonable" cost (which might not necessarily be the lowest cost).

cost-effectiveness analysis   The comparison of the cost-benefit ratios for the same service provided by different methods or with different equipment.

cost-per-case management   The method (philosophy) of hospital management in which hospitals try to control the costs for each kind of case so that the revenue for that case will cover the cost. Cost-per-case management is a new style of management which was developed when hospital revenue changed from reimbursement for services rendered to prospectively determined prices for various kinds of services. This change in reimbursement, in turn, came from the adoption of the prospective payment system (PPS) in the Medicare program. Previously, hospitals simply had to ensure that the aggregate of income covered the aggregate of costs.

cost-plus contract   See *cost-plus contract* under *contract*.

Cost Quality Management System (CQMS)   A system which merges clinical and financial data, patient-by-patient, in a hospital. The diagnosis and procedure data are standardized by use of the International Classification of Diseases, 9th Revision, Clinical Modification (ICD-9-CM), while the financial data are standardized by use of the International Classification of Clinical Services (ICCS). The system is intended to facilitate data display for the individual hospital and also to permit valid comparisons among institutions and services through reference to the database maintained by the Commission on Professional and Hospital Activities (CPHA). CQMS is a joint venture between CPHA and Arthur Andersen & Company.

cost-sharing   Out-of-pocket payment by patients for part of the cost of benefits of an insurance plan. The term is not properly applied to sharing in the cost of the insurance premium; it applies only to deductibles, coinsurance, and copayments.

cost-shifting   Increasing the charges to one group of patients (such as private pay patients, who presumably have the ability to pay) when the payment for another group of patients will not cover the costs for that group. If the government pays too little for its beneficiaries, for example, through the prospective payment system (PPS), it is clear that the cost will be shifted to other payers.

cost-to-charge ratio   See *cost-to-charge ratio* under *ratio*.

coupler   See *problem-knowledge coupler*.

coverage   In health care reform discussions, "coverage" is most often used to describe the group of people for whom health insurance is available, rather than the particular services paid for (see *benefits* and *insurance coverage*). For example, coverage may be for senior citizens (as a part of Medicare), for those persons who opt to purchase Medicare supplement insurance, for employees of a given company, and so on. In the health care reform movement, "universal coverage" is a goal:

covered person   See *enrollee*.

CPI   See *consumer price index (CPI)* under *index (numerical)*.

CPT   Current Procedural Terminology. See *Physicians' Current Procedural Terminology*.

credentialing   A term used to describe the process of determining eligibility for hospital medical staff membership, and privileges to be granted, to physicians and other professionals in the light of their academic preparation, licensing, training, and performance. Privileges are granted by the hospital's governing body, ordinarily upon recommendation of the medical staff, usually via the medical staff's credentials committee. (The exact procedure for "credentialing" is delineated in the hospital or medical staff bylaws.) The governing body must first verify the physician's credentials and determine whether they are adequate for admission to the medical staff. The governing body must then decide the more difficult question of what privileges the individual shall be granted initially and, upon periodic review of the professional's credentials and performance, whether it is necessary to modify them. Credentials and performance are periodically reviewed, and medical staff membership (and/or privileges) may be denied, modified, or withdrawn.

centralized credentialing   Credentialing of physicians by an organization outside a hospital, either non-profit or private. A single application from a physician will serve for all the hospitals participating in the service. The hospitals also share disciplinary information.

credentials committee   A committee of the medical staff charged with reviewing the credentials and performance of physicians and making recommendations as to medical staff membership and clinical privileges to be granted or modified.

critical path   A statement of what steps and procedures should be carried out for the diagnostic evaluation of a patient or for the management (treatment) for a given diagnosis or problem, and the optimum sequence with which they should be carried out. The term comes from the Critical Path Method (CPM), which is similar to the Program Evaluation and Review Technique (PERT), first described in connection with project management procedures developed during World War II. CPM is called a project network technique, it is typically developed with the aid of a computer, and is graphically displayed as a sort of road map.
  A major influence toward the use of CPM in medical care was the emergence of teams for taking care of patients, and the communication problems which ensued (there was less need for coordination when medical care involved only the one physician). The goal of critical paths is to insure that (only) the indicated steps are taken, that they are taken in the correct sequence, and distributed over the shortest time consonant with high quality of care. As a result, the quality of care should be optimal and the cost minimal. Because resources vary from hospital to hospital, critical paths are usually produced locally, in contrast with clinical practice guidelines, which generally come from authoritative bodies. Also called clinical care paths.

Current Procedural Terminology (CPT)   See *Physicians' Current Procedural Terminology*.

current ratio   See *current ratio* under *ratio*.

custodial   Pertains to watching over and protecting, rather than, in the health care field, attempting to provide treatment.

customary fee   See *customary, prevailing, reasonable charge (or fee) (CPR)*.

customary, prevailing, reasonable charge (or fee) (CPR)   The charge (1) or "fee" (same as charge), usually of a physician, which has traditionally been defined as that charge which is the lowest of the following: the actual charge made for the service; the physician or supplier's "customary" (usual) charge for the service; or the fee "prevailing" in the community for the service. Such fees vary according to specialty, geographic area, and the physician's charge system. Increases in such fees are typically limited by economic indexes (see *index (numerical)*) imposed by the paying agency. The definition of "reasonable and customary charge (or fee)" is under scrutiny by the federal government with the idea that the fees should be "inherently" reasonable, that is, related to some real worth of the service rather than a comparison. The Tax Equity and Fiscal Responsibility Act (TEFRA) and Medicare regulations both give specific formulas for calculating the "reasonable charges" limitation on physician fees. Synonym(s): customary fee, prevailing fee, and Usual, Customary and Reasonable (UCR).

customer   In health care, "customer" is often used to mean the person or entity buying the services. For example, an employer might be the customer of a health care plan which enrolls the employees. In the context of quality management, the customer is the person (or department) for whom services are provided. For example, the customers of the clinical laboratory include not only the patient, but the physician who receives the lab results, and perhaps the accounting department which must determine the charges. An important process in quality improvement is to determine who the customers are, what they need, and whether these needs are being met. See also *consumer*.

cybernaut   A "traveller" in cyberspace.

cyberspace   Computer-generated space, in which the traveller is called a "cybernaut." The term was coined by science fiction author William Gibson in 1984. It is now also being applied to computer conferencing, computer bulletin boards, and other innovative communication activities and applications of information technology, particularly in education and health care. An example: a college course is sometimes said to be conducted in cyberspace when it is carried out primarily or largely with an electronic network rather than in a classroom. Students in such a course may be employed in widely separated sites, and the faculty member may address them informally in the electronic network from wherever she happens to be. The reference library is, of course, electronic. Questions, answers, and student and faculty discussion may be posted on the class's computer bulletin board at any time by students or faculty. In addition, scheduled interactive "class periods" for the dispersed faculty and students are held.

D

daily service charge Same as *room rate*; see under *rate (charge)*.

damages A legal term describing the money to be paid to a plaintiff by the defendant when the defendant is found to be liable. The term "damages" is sometimes used more restrictively to describe the monetary value of the plaintiff's injuries, property loss, and the like.

Darling case A landmark hospital law case which established that the hospital is responsible for care provided to patients, and that the medical staff must be accountable to the hospital for the care provided by medical staff members. The case involved a young man named Darling who was brought to a hospital with a leg fracture suffered while playing football. Through a series of events (notably, lack of communication among nurses, doctors, and hospital, and failure by the hospital and medical staff to enforce their own bylaws) the patient's leg became gangrenous and was eventually lost. *Darling v. Charleston Community Memorial Hospital*, 33 Ill.2d 326, 211 N.E.2d 253 (1965), *cert. denied*, 383 U.S. 946 (1966).

data Material, facts, or figures on which discussion is held or from which inferences are drawn or decisions made. A distinction is sometimes made between "data" and "information"; generally, data have to be somehow "digested" (manipulated, summarized, organized, or interpreted) in order to become information. No rigid standardization in terminology has appeared in this regard, although generally the term "information" is rarely applied to material which is "raw."

database A collection of data or information organized with some type of structure, such as records (rows) and fields (columns). A database record is group of items of information logically connected in some fashion. Records are often subdivided into smaller units of data known as data elements or "fields." For example, a telephone book is a database (collection) of data records, each listing being one record. Each record in the telephone book might be further subdivided into three data elements or fields: name, address, and telephone number.

Database also describes a type of software application or language used to store and manipulate such data on computer systems. When referring to computer databases, they may be further described by being hierarchical or relational, for instance. See *database management system*.

clinical database The array of information (data set) about a patient which is collected by the physician and others caring for the patient in order to make a diagnosis and to be able to detect changes in the patient's condition during treatment.

statistical database A compilation of data about a number of events (illnesses, for example) or objects (patients, for example) which has as its purpose the description of the group of events or objects. For example, a statistical database consisting of identical items of information about many patients who smoke gives a statistical description of smokers, and is used to estimate the risk of smoking, an element in health risk appraisal.

database management system (DBMS) A computer program used to manage a database. In its simplest form, it is a computerized filing system. In more elaborate forms, it relates information from different files together to produce new files, reports, and detailed analyses. Different DBMSs also tend to have their own languages with which they can be programmed for specific purposes, such as automatically performing certain functions when certain types of data are entered. The actual DBMS is frequently hidden from the user by a "user-friendly interface" which prompts and guides the user every step of the way. DBMSs may be further described as being hierarchical or relational, for instance. See also *Structured Query Language (SQL)*.

data element In general usage, an "item of information." When used in connection with computers, a data element may be one part of a data record (a logically connected group of data elements). Synonym(s): field. See also, *database*.

data set A specified set of items of information. The data set for a person's address, for example, may be name, street address, city, state, and ZIP code. In the hospital, the term "data set" would be applied, for example, to a discharge abstract (see *abstract*) and to a patient's bill. In this illustration, the nucleus of both data sets is, at a minimum, the Uniform Hospital Discharge Data Set (UHDDS) specified by the federal government (see below).

patient's data set A computer record of selected data items about an episode of care, including identity of the patient, identity of the physician, dates of care, diagnoses, procedures, reference to the original medical record, and other information.

Uniform Hospital Discharge Data Set (UHDDS) The items of medical record information required by the federal government as the medical content of the patient's bill under Medicare. Assignment to a Diagnosis Related Group (DRG) is made from this data set by the fiscal intermediary. UHDDS contains, among other data, patient age, sex, and up to five diagnoses and four procedures. Both diagnoses and procedures are expressed not in words but in the numerical category codes of the International Classification of Disease, Ninth Revision, Clinical Modification (ICD-9-CM).

data repository See *data warehouse*.

data standards See *hospital electronic medical data standards*.

data warehouse An emerging component of integrated computer systems. The data warehouse obtains data from one or more sources and makes it readily available for answering management questions about the organization and its activities. In the hospital, transactions such as patient billing, collecting insurance payments, giving services to patients, purchasing, and others are going on continuously, and access to this flowing stream of data "on-line" in order to obtain management information is awkward and costly. An "off-line" data warehouse system: (1) takes periodic (daily, weekly, monthly) "snapshots" of the computer records coming from these transactions, (2) retains only the data elements of each transaction which are needed for management information (to reduce the bulk of the data and speed the access to it), (3) formats the data in such a fashion that the data from different sources can be handled by the computer as though they were from a single source, (4) stores the data with an eye to ease of access, and (5) provides tools (computer systems) by which the data can be interrogated.

A data warehouse would probably be classified as a "value-added" component of a data system, since it stores and transfers data. The resulting database (or set of relational databases) may be within the hospital or off-site, if the data warehouse operation serves a number of hospitals. A multi-hospital data warehouse not only may offer economies of scale, but it also offers a unique opportunity for exchange of information—governed, of course, by strict security measures for the preservation of confidentiality as to patients, physicians, and institutions. Also called a data repository.

decision support software (DSS) A special class of computer software designed to make relevant knowledge accessible to decision makers. In health care, DSS falls into three classes, depending on who is the intended decision maker:

1) Reference DSS. For physicians and other professionals there are indexing tools which significantly improve access to published literature and the information it contains. Literature is typically organized around diseases, injuries, and proce-dures rather than the problems presented by patients, so these tools facilitate the traditional practice of medicine in which the professional is the authority and the patient is the passive recipient of care. They may also cite probabilities for various diagnoses and success of various treatments for the *typical*, rather than *specific*, patient.

2) Lay education DSS. For consumers there is a fast-growing array of popular software and there are numerous informal networks on the information highway (in cyberspace).

3) Guidance DSS. For joint use by the professional caregiver and the patient there is DSS which presents the current information from the literature in a manner understandable by both professional and lay person. The goal of this software is the elimination of knowledge asymmetry between the two. It eliminates the necessity for the professional to rely on memorized information, insures complete-ness of knowledge, and provides guidance for shared decision making (SDM) and truly informed consent.

deductible The amount of money an insured person must pay "at the front end" before the insurer will pay. In automobile collision insurance with a $100 deductible, the insured must pay any damage under $100 in its entirety, and the first $100 when the total is over that amount. The reason for introducing this concept into health care coverage is primarily to discourage "unnecessary" use of services, and also to reduce insurance premiums, since all claims have a minimum amount which the insurer will be spared on every claim. Health plans have developed two other types of "front end" payments: see *coinsurance* and *copayment*.

defensive medicine   The obtaining of services, mainly diagnostic procedures, in anticipation of defending against a possible lawsuit by the person treated alleging malpractice. The primary reasons for obtaining the services is to avoid having to defend against a contention that omission of a test was negligent medical care, and to show the jury in a malpractice trial documented evidence that other possibilities were "ruled out" by the tests.

Ordinarily, diagnostic tests are obtained because the physician honestly needs the information they provide. In defensive medicine, however, the tests have little or no medical value. For example, a physician may be quite satisfied that a sprained ankle is just that; nevertheless, because of the threat of a malpractice suit, she may still obtain an X-ray in order to have evidence that she did not overlook a fracture.

definitive care   A level of therapeutic intervention capable of providing comprehensive health care services for a specific condition.

deinstitutionalization   The discharge of mental patients from mental institutions, with continued care to be provided in the community. This movement was made possible by the development of psychotropic drugs, which modify a patient's behavior to such an extent that she is considered able to function within the community.

demarketing   Efforts to persuade individuals not to buy, or to go elsewhere. A hospital has a serious problem when the price set for a given Diagnosis Related Group (DRG) under the prospective payment system (PPS) is lower than the lowest cost the hospital can achieve for care for a patient with that DRG and still maintain quality. Under those circumstances, the hospital may elect to discontinue caring for such patients (for example, pediatrics). Alternatively, it may develop some more subtle strategy to discourage patients with a problem which falls into the DRG from coming to that hospital, or to discourage physicians from bringing such patients. The latter efforts have been labelled "demarketing."

democratization   A process of putting more decision-making into the hands of the individual. A system of health care in which persons collaborate in the decisions about their health and health care is a democratized system.

demographic data   The class of information about a person which includes such items as age, sex, race, income, marital status, and education. Demographic data is important for proper patient care, and is also used as the data with which to compile certain statistics (demographics) on a population, for example, in the study of the distribution of certain types of injuries and illnesses.

demographics   Descriptions of patient populations or service area populations in such terms as age, sex, race, educational level, income, family size, and ethnic background.

Department of Health and Human Services (DHHS)   The department of the executive branch of the federal government responsible for the federal health programs in the civilian sector, and for Social Security. DHHS is the portion of the Department of Health, Education, and Welfare (DHEW) left after the establishment of the Department of Education as an separate department. DHHS is sometimes referred to as HHS.

Department of Justice (DOJ)   The federal government department which enforces certain federal laws; for example, antitrust laws. The Department of Justice is headed by the United States Attorney General.

Department of Transportation (DOT)   The department in the executive branch of the federal government which is concerned with transportation. One concern of DOT is emergency medical services.

development   See *fund-raising*.

Diagnosis Related Group (DRG)   A hospital patient classification system developed under federal grants at Yale University. The current payment system for Medicare is based on the federal government's setting a predetermined price for the "package of care" in the hospital (exclusive of physician's fees) required for each DRG. If the hospital can provide the care for less than the DRG price, it can keep the difference; if the care costs the hospital more than the price, the hospital has to absorb the difference. Originally each DRG was intended to contain patients who were roughly the same kind of patients in a medical sense and who spent about the same amount of time in the hospital. The groupings were subsequently redefined so that, in addition to medical similarity, resource consumption (ancillary services, see *service*, as well as inpatient service days) was approximately the same within a given group. There are now 468 DRGs identified on the basis of the following criteria: the principal diagnosis (the final diagnosis which, after study in the hospital, was determined to be chiefly responsible for the hospitalization); whether an operating room procedure (see *procedure*) was performed; the patient's age; comorbidity (see *morbidity*); and complications.

A number of efforts are underway to modify DRGs by the use of severity of illness measures, and to develop new DRGs for specific classes of patients, as in the case of pediatrics with development of Pediatric-Modified Diagnosis Related Groups (PM-DRGs). See also *prospective payment system (PPS)* and *Ambulatory Patient Group (APG)*.

Pediatric-Modified Diagnosis Related Groups (PM-DRGs)   Diagnosis Related Groups (DRGs) for the classification of pediatric medical conditions. PM-DRGs have been developed by the National Association of Children's Hospitals and Related Institutions, Inc. (NACHRI) in a research project funded by the Health Care Financing Administration (HCFA). They add about 100 DRGs to the current DRG system. PM-DRGs are for use when a prospective payment system (PPS) is to be used for pediatric patients, and also by hospitals in analysis of utilization-management activities, study of pediatric case mix, and pricing of services.

Diagnostic and Therapeutic Technology Assessment (DATTA) Program   A program of the American Medical Association (AMA) for assessing medical technology, with the purpose of providing authoritative information to physicians on the appropriate use of specific medical technology.

diagnostic cost groups (DCGs)   A system for paying for hospital care being tried by the Health Care Financing Administration (HCFA) for patients of Medicare HMOs (see *health maintenance organization (HMO)*). In this system, a patient's prior hospitalization history during the preceding 15 months is used to predict future costs.

Prior utilization is expected to reflect the patient's health status and the physician's practice patterns. Each patient is placed in one of eight DCGs, depending on costliness, with the higher number DCGs reflecting higher expected costs to treat the patient. For each DCG, there is a set of cost weights that depend on the patient's age, sex, and welfare status. A formula results in the setting of the HMO's capitation rate.

dietary risk factors   Eating patterns which increase the likelihood for developing disease or other adverse health effects. Examples are: percentage of fat calories above 30 percent of total food calories increase one's risk for death from heart disease; being overweight is linked to heart disease, cancer, and diabetes; lack of adequate fluid intake puts many elderly persons at risk of dehydration.

digital   When used to describe information (data), "digital" means based on a system of discrete steps, such as counting the fingers on one's hand. Frequently, the term "digital" is associated with binary logic, where each bit of information can have one of two states (such as "on" or "off," or "true" or "false"). This term can also describe most computers in use today, which process information in this manner. "Digital" is distinguished from "analog," which treats information as based on a continuum, such as body temperature. In order to convert analog information to digital information, one must arbitrarily select samples (steps) along the continuum, and discard the rest of the information.

direct care provider   An individual who is responsible for the care of an individual, as contrasted with a "consultant" who is responsible only for giving an opinion. However, the consultant may take over the care of the patient and become the direct care provider.

direct contract   An agreement between an employer (or health plan or insurer) and a health care provider for the provision of health care services to the employees (beneficiaries). This is often referred to as a "direct provider agreement (DPA)."

directive   See *advance directive*.

director (governance)   A member of the governing body when the official term for that body is "board of directors." When the governing body is called the "board of trustees," its members are individually "trustees."

director (management)   An operating officer. The title "director" is used by many institutions for their officers and executives. The chief executive officer (CEO) may be called *the* director, and various subordinates may carry titles such as "director of development," "director of nursing," and the like.

director of medical affairs (DMA)   The person designated by the governing body to be responsible for management of the medical staff and for carrying out policy for the medical staff as promulgated by the board. Ordinarily the DMA is a physician, and may be nominated by the medical staff. A physician with this title is ordinarily paid. This term is discussed further under *chief of staff*.

director of nursing   See *nursing service administrator*.

direct provider agreement (DPA)   An agreement between an employer, an HMO, or other health care plan and a health care provider for the provision of health care services to the enrollees.

disability   The absence or loss of physical, mental, or emotional function and, sometimes, earning ability. May be temporary or permanent, total or partial. "Disability" will have a specific legal definition for a particular purpose; for example, Social Security or workers' compensation laws.

disaster   A sudden natural or man-made event which causes extensive damage, destruction, or injury, and requires mobilization of emergency health care resources. Examples are fire, flood, earthquake, tornado, collapse of a building, nuclear accident, war, mine cave-in, airplane crash.

disaster medical assistance team (DMAT)   A team capable of stabilizing casualties, using advanced trauma life support (ATLS) methods (life support), sorting (triage), and evacuation. DMATs are a part of the National Disaster Medical System (NDMS). Several DMATs are organized into a clearing and staging unit (CSU).

disaster plan   See *disaster preparedness plan.*

disaster preparedness plan   A formal plan for coping with a disaster. An accredited hospital is expected to have both an external disaster plan and an internal disaster plan (see below). Often such plans have basic elements relating to any kind of disaster and dealing with such items as emergency communication, alerting of police and fire departments, mobilization of off-duty personnel, and the like. The basic plan also has supplements for various kinds of disasters; for example, a nuclear disaster would call for different procedures than a flood or a tornado. It is expected that the written plan will periodically be tested and modified on the basis of disaster drills. Synonym(s): disaster plan.

> **external disaster plan**   A formal disaster preparedness plan for coping with a disaster in the community, or for which the hospital may be expected to provide health care services.

> **internal disaster plan**   A formal disaster preparedness plan for coping with a disaster, such as a fire or hazardous materials, within the institution itself.

disbursement   Paying money to take care of an expense or a debt.

discharge   The formal release of a patient from a physician's care or from a hospital (in Canada, a hospital discharge is called a "separation"). Sometimes called "signing out" the patient. A discharge terminates certain responsibilities on the part of the provider. There are several kinds of discharge:

discharge planning   The process of making sure that arrangements are made outside the hospital to receive the patient upon discharge and to provide the necessary continuity of care.

disease   An illness or disorder of the function of the body or of certain tissues, organs, or systems. Diseases differ from injuries in that injuries are the result of external physical or chemical agents.

acute disease A disease which normally is of short duration—a rule of thumb is 30 days or less—and which ordinarily is confined to a single episode.

chronic disease A disease which requires more than one episode of care, or is of long duration (more than 30 days, for example), or both.

disincentive An undesirable "reward" for undesired behavior. For example, as part of efforts to reduce hospital and physician costs, patients are sometimes required to pay the first dollars for services; this payment may be a deductible, copayment, or coinsurance. The deductibles are a "disincentive" (a negative incentive) to seek the care, and thus an incentive to be frugal.

disproportionate share hospital (DSH) A Medicare term for a hospital serving a higher than average proportion of low-income patients.

dispute resolution See *alternative dispute resolution (ADR)*.

diversification A term coming into use as hospitals enter lines of business other than care of the sick and injured in an effort to obtain revenue from a variety of sources and remain solvent. The hospital is typically restructured in the process of diversification, and foundations, holding companies, and the like may result. The new "businesses" may be other health care enterprises such as home care or neighborhood health centers; they may also be other activities, such as offering its collection or public relations services to other clients.

divestiture Getting rid of something, for example, to comply with a court order breaking up a monopoly. A corporate sale of a subsidiary corporation (see *corporation*) is said to be a divestiture.

divide and dump To separate high-risk from low-risk employees and "dump" (not insure) the high-risk employees.

divided standard of medical care See *standard of care (medical)*.

DNS See *Domain Name System*.

do not resuscitate order (DNR) An order by the physician, with respect to a specific patient, to the effect that, should cardiac arrest or respiratory arrest occur, no attempt should be made to give cardiopulmonary resuscitation (CPR) to the patient (restart the heart or otherwise revive her). "Do not resuscitate" is sometimes translated into the jargon that the patient is "not to be coded," or "do not code this patient"; this means that a code blue signal should not be issued. A suggestion has been made that the term "do not resuscitate" be changed to "do not attempt resuscitation" (DNAR). A DNR order may be issued for one or more of three reasons: (1) no medical benefit; (2) poor quality of life predicted after CPR; or (3) poor quality of life before CPR. Or, such an order may be issued because a competent adult patient has asked not to be resuscitated. There is controversy about the circumstances under which a DNR order may be issued for an incompetent patient. The conservative approach is to obtain the consent of the patient's legal representative for any DNR order; however, some believe that no consent is required where there is no medical benefit, since CPR would not be medically indicated under these circumstances. (For example, consent is not required to "not perform" an appendectomy, if an appendectomy is not medically indicated.) Synonym(s): not to be coded, do not code, no-code order, order not to resuscitate (ONTR), do not attempt resuscitation (DNAR).

doc-in-a-box A slang term for any one of a growing variety of ambulatory care facilities: storefront physician's offices or clinics; walk-in outpatient facilities; or specialized offices for foot care, dietary advice, and the like. The term is less likely to be used for ambulatory surgical centers, sports medicine centers, and other similar facilities with more formal structure, and which offer continuity of care.

Dole Foundation for the Employment of People with Disabilities A foundation based in Washington, DC, established by Senator Robert Dole, to make grants to community-based nonprofit organizations for innovative programs for job-skill training and job placement for people with disabilities.

Domain Name System (DNS) An addressing method used by the Internet that allows words a human can recognize, like "tringa.com", to represent a unique network address that only a machine can love, like "198.87.128.43". These numerical addresses, fitting into a pattern ranging from 0.0.0.0 to 255.255.255.255, are referred to as "Internet Protocol (IP)" addresses. Like any computer network system, each computer or other resource on the network must have an exact and unique address. When the network is worldwide, like the Internet, and connects millions of computers, some system must be enforced to maintain these unique addresses. The organization fulfilling this responsibility is Network Solutions, Inc. (NSI), previously the Internet Network Information Center (InterNIC). Whenever someone wishes to add a resource to the Internet, such as adding a site (home page) to the World-Wide Web (WWW), they must obtain a unique address from NSI. Traditionally this has been done by applying for a domain name, like tringa.com, which is then linked to a unique numerical (IP) address. Both the domain name and the IP address must be unique, and are assigned by NSI on a "first come, first served" basis. This address is also referred to as the resource's "Uniform Resource Locator (URL)", particularly when the address contains the domain name plus the name and location of the file referred to, and the protocol to be used to *download* (or read, or browse) the file.

  A current policy statement for registering domain names with NSI is located at the following URL: "ftp://rs.internic.net/policy/internic/internic-domain-1.txt". For a discussion of the context for DNS, see *Internet*.

donated services The estimated monetary value of the services rendered by personnel who receive no monetary compensation or only partial monetary compensation for their services. The term is applied to services rendered by members of religious orders, societies, volunteers, and similar groups.

download Downloading, and its counterpart "uploading", refer to the transfer of data between two computers. The data, usually in the format of one or more files, is uploaded to or downloaded from the other computer. Either computer may be referred to as being the "local" or the "remote" machine, depending on your location. One of the two computers is typically operating in an unattended mode, and is then referred to as the "host", while the other may be referred to as the "client", although these roles may be easily reversed. One way to remember the distinction between up and downloading is to think of data files as books you either "put up" or "get down" from a shelf.

DPA See *direct provider agreement*.

DRG cost weight A number, or weight, assigned to each Diagnosis Related Group (DRG) by the federal government. It reflects the DRG's use of resources in relation to the cost of the average Medicare patient as determined by the federal government. The average Medicare patient's cost, when multiplied by the DRG cost weight, gives the price for the DRG in question.

DRG creep A change in the distribution of patients among Diagnosis Related Groups (DRGs) without a real change in the distribution of patients treated in the hospital. It is feared that hospitals and physicians will change their record-keeping and reporting so that more patients will appear in higher-priced DRGs, and thus hospital income will be increased without a corresponding increase in cost—the creep will be "upward," and will represent exploitation of the payment system. This term is sometimes inappropriately used when the fact of the matter is that the apparent creep simply represents a systematic improvement in record-keeping and coding. When this is the case, of course, there should be a one-time adjustment, which the PPS system should recognize as laudable. Sometimes called "code creep".

DRG enhancer A computer program that arranges the medical data for billing to Medicare so as to achieve the best Diagnosis Related Group (DRG) classification, i.e., the one with the biggest price tag.

DRG payment system Originally, slang for the prospective payment system (PPS) of Medicare. However, this term may now be appropriate usage when payment by other than the Medicare program (insurance plans, for example) is also based on Diagnosis Related Groups (DRGs).

DRG-specific price blending See *price blending*.

DRG system See *prospective payment system (PPS)*.

drug utilization A term which usually refers to the patterns of use of drugs by individual physicians and in hospitals. The term "drug utilization" usually occurs in connection with the terms "drug utilization committee" or "drug utilization study," both of which have to do with efforts to determine whether certain drugs are used appropriately (for example, whether obsolete drugs are still being given, or whether certain drugs, such as antibiotics, are given for the correct indications).

DSH See *disproportionate share hospital*.

Duke Activity Status Index (DASI) See *Duke Activity Status Index (DASI)* under *quality of life scale*.

dumping The denial or limitation of the provision of medical care to, or the transfer elsewhere of, patients who are not able to pay or for which the payment method (for example, the prospective payment system (PPS)) does not pay the hospital enough to cover its costs. Laws intended to prevent dumping typically prohibit the transfer of patients if the transfer cannot be justified by medical necessity. Synonym(s): patient dumping, case shifting.

granny dumping The practice of abandoning an ill, elderly, indigent person at a hospital or other health care facility.

durable medical equipment (DME) Medical equipment, such as a wheelchair, breathing equipment, home dialysis equipment, or other equipment, that is prescribed by the physician. The term is used most often when DME is used in the home.

E

Early and Periodic Screening Diagnosis and Treatment Program (EPSDT) A program required of states by Medicaid for children under age 21 in families receiving Aid to Families with Dependent Children (AFDC). EPSDT is designed to detect physical and mental defects and arrange treatment.

early offer See *early offer* under *alternative dispute resolution (ADR)*.

economic index See *economic index* under *index*.

economic system The way in which goods and services are produced, distributed, and consumed. In health care, the traditional provider-driven system is moving toward a market-driven system.

market-driven system An economic system which responds to the demands of the market, that is, those of the purchaser. The term is currently being applied in health care with the emergence of competitive health care delivery plans which seek to attract "customers" by offering (1) more of what the customers want (amenities as well as services) or (2) attractive prices (that is, price competition). Note that the customer is the person paying for the service, and is not necessarily the consumer (the patient).

provider-driven system An economic system in which providers (in health care, physicians, other professionals, and institutions), "prescribe" and furnish those services which they consider to be the best care for the patients. Such a system is intended to meet the needs of the patients as determined by the providers rather than to meet the demands of the purchasers of care.

education The acquisition of knowledge and skills; see also *training*.

health education Education which is directed at increasing the information of individuals and populations, especially communities, about health and its maintenance and the prevention of disease and injury; bringing about modifications in the behavior of individuals so as to achieve better health; and changing social policy in the direction of a more healthful environment and practices.

patient education   Teaching patients what they need to know about their illness or condition, especially how to care for themselves.

effectiveness   The degree to which the effort expended, or the action taken, achieves the desired effect (result or objective). For example, one drug is more effective than another if it relieves certain symptoms to a greater extent, or in a higher proportion of patients. See also *efficiency*, which is often confused with effectiveness. Synonym(s): efficacy.

efficacy   See *effectiveness*.

efficiency   The relationship of the amount of work accomplished to the amount of effort required. A given hospital's food service is more efficient than another hospital's in one measure if, for example, it can furnish meals to patients for a lower average cost per meal (assuming that the meals are of equal quality). Although efficiency is usually thought of in terms of cost, it can equally well be measured in other ways, such as time; for example, the automobile racing crew which can change a set of tires in the shortest time is the most efficient. See also *effectiveness*, which is often confused with efficiency.

elder care   Home care of the elderly by relatives. Tax relief for families who provide home health care for an elderly relative has been proposed. Relief has also been proposed for families who care for a dependent suffering from Alzheimer's disease.

elective   A term that refers to treatment which is medically advisable, but not critical. Elective care (such as hospitalization, treatment, or surgery) can be scheduled in advance, in contrast to emergency care, which must be rendered immediately to avoid death or serious disability. See *elective surgery* under *surgery (treatment)*.

electronic data interchange (EDI)   The exchange of routine business transactions via computer. EDI enforces a level of standardization in the way the electronically transmitted data is formatted, making it possible for a variety of different computer system to exchange data. The term is used in health care primarily in connection with claims and other financial transactions. Approximately 200 vendors offer products in this field.

electronic medical record (EMR)   See *medical record*.

eligibility   A term usually used in health care with reference to whether an individual may be enrolled in a given insurance plan, governmental program, or other health care plan. Also may refer to the qualification of a health care plan to contract with HCFA to provide services to Medicare beneficiaries.

eligibility period   The period of time a new employee has to sign up for life or health insurance without having to take a physical examination or otherwise show insurability. After the eligibility period has expired, the employee may be denied insurance because of a preexisting condition, or have to pay higher premiums.

e-mail "Electronic mail". This is used to describe a variety of messages that are not only transmitted electronically, but are intended to be read and replied to electronically as well. Consequently, e-mail does not include faxes, telegrams, or other such messages which are transmitted electronically but routinely presented to the receiver as 'hard copy' (paper).

emergency A situation requiring immediate attention in order to prevent death or severe disability. A situation less critical is "urgent." The least critical level is "elective."

emergency medical technician (EMT) An allied health professional with special training in on-site and in-transit care of injured and emergency medical patients (victims), and also in providing emergency care in the hospital emergency department (ED) if requested to. State regulations typically govern the use of specific titles for EMTs, the training required for each of several levels, supplementary training needed for special procedures (such as the administration of intravenous fluids, the insertion of a tube into a patient's airway for assistance in breathing, the use of cardiac defibrillation equipment, and the like). In national usage, there are three levels of EMTs, depending on training:

employee A person who works for and is paid by another (the employer), and who is under the control of the employer. An employee is to be distinguished from an independent contractor, who works for himself. The line between the two is often fuzzy, but the legal consequences are important. Different tests to determine whether someone is an employee or independent contractor are used for different purposes—taxes, workers' compensation, liability, unemployment insurance, and so forth. The same person can easily be both an employee and an independent contractor, at the same time, for different purposes.

employee assistance program (EAP) An occupational health service program to help employees with substance abuse or physical or behavioral problems deal with these problems when they affect job performance. The assistance may be provided within the organization or by referral to outside resources.

employee health benefit plan An organization's plan for health benefits for its employees and their dependents. The term generally refers to the "package" of benefits which are provided. Such plans are among the "fringe benefits" of the employees, and thus are not part of the employee's salary. The employees may or may not contribute to paying the cost by deductions from their salaries.

employee health service A service provided by an organization to examine persons prior to employment and to give certain health care (and, often, counseling) to employees.

Employee Retirement Income Security Act (ERISA) A 1974 federal act which prevents states from regulating self-insured employers. It also had provisions requiring health plans to provide certain information to enrollees.

employment at will Employment of an individual without a personal or union contract. Notwithstanding the lack of an employment contract, however, termination of such an employee under certain circumstances may subject an employer to liability for "wrongful discharge." Such circumstances include a discharge violating an implied contract, not carried out in "good faith and fair dealing," or against public policy. For example, firing an employee who reasonably refuses to do something dangerous may be against public policy.

empowerment   See *patient empowerment*.

encounter   The personal contact between the patient and a professional health care giver. This term is typically used only with respect to personnel involved in assessment or treatment, or providing social services, not with obtaining a prescription drug from a pharmacy, for example.

end-stage renal disease (ESRD)   Renal (kidney) disease in which the kidneys no longer function enough to sustain life, a condition known as renal insufficiency. Life may be sustained by kidney transplant in some instances, or by hemodialysis (see *dialysis*). Specific benefits are available for patients with ESRD under Medicare, which is the primary source for paying for long-term hemodialysis, either in the hospital or in the home.

energy agent   See *energy agent* under *agent*.

enrollee   As used in health insurance and with prepayment plans, a person who is covered (receives benefits) under a contract for care. Sometimes called "member" or "covered person". See also *subscriber*.

entrepreneur   A person who organizes a new venture and assumes the risk. This is in contrast with the new term "intrapreneur," meaning a person *within* an organization who creates a new venture or "product" for the organization.

entropy prevention   The set of management activities directed at maintaining quality and enthusiasm in the performance of established activities and duties which are not in need of change. Entropy is a term taken from physics for the tendency of any system (process) to lose energy, to "run down," if no additional energy is provided. An appreciable amount of management energy is applied to change which, while resisted, is seen as "where the action is." However, an equal or even greater amount of management energy must be applied to keep ongoing activities (systems) interesting and exciting, and to prevent quality from declining and change from occurring.

environmental assessment   A technique used in planning in which influences and events external to the organization which are felt likely to present either problems or opportunities are listed. An attempt is then made to predict the effects of these factors on the organization, and to suggest the appropriate responses. It is to be contrasted with "environmental impact," in which the effects of actions of the organization on its environment are assessed.

epidemiology   The study of diseases or causes of disease in relationship to a population, such as a hospital or a community. Epidemiology deals primarily with the analysis of existing data rather than data collected prospectively in an experimental design.

episode   A series of events which is distinct in itself. For example, a period of fever which disappears may be an episode of fever within a continuous process, such as a chronic illness.

episode of care   A continuous course of care by a hospital or physician for a specific medical problem or condition. Often the term has a specific definition under a federal or state statute.

equity (access)   Fairness. This is one great impetus to health care reform; inequities among regions of the country, between rural and urban settings, among ethnic groups, and among socioeconomic groups, in access to and quality of both preventive and curative services, are widely reported.

equity (finance)   Assets minus liabilities; also called "net worth." See *asset* and *liability (financial)*.

Estes Park Institute (EPI)   An independent nonprofit corporation providing education and other services for the health care community. EPI's main programs are national conferences for hospital medical staff officers, hospital and other health care administrator and trustees, and their spouses.

Eutaw Group   An ad hoc health care "think tank" with William F. Bridgers, MD, as Head. Bridgers is founding Dean of the School of Public Health of the University of Alabama. The Eutaw Group contends that the health care universe is one comprised of "haves" and "havenots," and that this distinction is more important than the usual distinction into urban and rural. As a result, the Eutaw Group proposes a community care plan as an alternative (or complement) to the accountable health plan (AHP) for the underserved populations, both urban and rural. Bridgers is the author of *Health Care Reform: A Dilemma and a Pathway for the Health Care System* (1992).

euthanasia   Permitting the death of a hopelessly ill or injured person (passive euthanasia), or causing the death of that individual in a reasonably painless manner (active euthanasia) as an act of mercy. The term "euthanasia" may be applied to the policy as well as to the act. The line between active and passive euthanasia is not always clear, and some believe that asserting the right to die (refusing or withdrawing life-sustaining treatment) on behalf of an incompetent individual is a form of euthanasia.

evaluation of care   Assessment of the degree to which care measures up to accepted standards.

excess coverage   See *excess coverage* under *insurance coverage*.

exclusive contract   See *exclusive contract* under *contract*.

exclusive dealing   An agreement between a seller and buyer, for the seller to sell only to the buyer (or the buyer to buy only from the seller). When such an arrangement unfavorably affects competition, it may violate the federal antitrust laws.

exclusive provider organization (EPO)   An alternative delivery system (ADS) for health care which is a cross between a health maintenance organization (HMO) and a preferred provider organization (PPO). As in PPOs, the providers are paid on a fee-for-service basis and generally the providers are not at risk. However, beneficiaries have less freedom in obtaining their care from providers outside the panel than they do in PPOs (where other providers may be employed by the patient, but at some financial penalty).

executive director   See *chief executive officer (CEO)*.

ex officio   Membership by virtue of holding a position or office. An ex officio member of a body (such as a board of directors or a committee) may or may not have authority to vote, depending on the bylaws of the body.

expenditure target   A goal for attempting to hold down the rate of growth in expenditures. Such a target may be mandated by law and limit the payments which may be made, for example, to a physician in a given year. One such target is the Medicare Volume Performance Standards (MVPS).

expense   The using up of an asset (as in depreciation), or the cost of providing services or making a product, during an accounting period. The subtraction of expenses from revenue gives the net income.

experience rating   See *rating*.

Experiment in Patient Injury Compensation (EPIC)   A project which started in 1995 in Utah which combines features of no-fault and enterprise liability systems for compensation for injuries sustained by patients in the health care system. The sponsorship of EPIC is the Utah Alliance for Health Care, a coalition of medical, hospital, business, labor, and other community organizations.

explicit   Specifically stated. For example, if there are conditions tied to one's income which state that nothing can be spent on travel, that is an *explicit* limitation. If there are no conditions, but the income will not permit both a vacation trip and painting the house, the necessity for choice (or establishing priorities) is *implicit*; it goes "naturally" with the idea of limited funds. In financing medical and hospital care, limited funds require choices as to how to spend them. In the past, the rationing of funds has been implicit, but some states are beginning to use explicit methods; see *Oregon plan*.

external independent review   See *review*.

extraordinary treatment   See *treatment*.

F

---

facility (institution)   A health care facility, which is any institution organized to provide ambulatory, inpatient, residential, or other health care.

faith organization   A generic term covering all religious organizations. Such organizations, which exist in all communities, have certain common features: they address sickness and health through education and service, they believe in feeding the hungry, clothing the naked, and healing the sick. Because of these attributes, faith organizations often provide effective and potent vehicles for health efforts. Synonym: faith community.

family birth center   A family-centered unit in the hospital where mothers with normal pregnancies may, if they wish, deliver their babies in a hospital, but in a homelike environment.

family care home (FCH)   A family residence which provides rest home care to a limited number of persons. Usually the number of persons who can be cared for is stipulated by law or regulations as, for example, six or fewer (a greater number of persons turns the facility into a "rest home" and places it under rest home licensure and supervision requirements). May also be called "adult foster home."

family planning   Efforts to determine the number of children and their spacing in a family by the use of birth control methods.

family-centered maternity/newborn care   An approach to maternity and newborn care which emphasizes the physical and social needs of the entire family— mother, baby, and the others.

Federal Employees Health Benefits Program (FEHBP, FEP)   A voluntary group health insurance program for federal employees.

Federal Register   The daily publication of the United States government in which federal administrative agencies officially publish their rules (including proposed rules subject to public comment).

Federal Trade Commission (FTC)   A federal agency which has jurisdiction over unfair and deceptive trade practices. Some such practices may violate the federal antitrust laws. The FTC was created in 1914 by the Federal Trade Commission Act (15 U.S.C. sec. 45 (1982)).

federalism   A form of association between organizations which are independent but which delegate certain common functions to a central body. The United States is a federation. There is increasing interest in forming local federations among health care providers and agencies in order to allow organizations and institutions to retain their identities and yet to avoid duplication and thus to meet the unique health care needs of the individual community in the most appropriate and economical fashion.

federally qualified HMO (FQHMO)   A health maintenance organization (HMO) that has applied for and received a designation by HCFA as being "federally qualified," which makes the HMO eligible to apply for a Medicare contract. The HMO must meet a number of requirements, which are stricter than those required for a competitive medical plan (CMP). A federally qualified HMO may offer more diverse products than a CMP.

fee   A charge for a service rendered.

fee-for-service (FFS)   A method of paying physicians and other health care providers in which each service (for example, a doctor's office visit or operation) carries a fee. The physician's income under this system is made up from the fees she collects for services. Alternative methods of income for physicians are: (1) a salary, such as one paid by a health maintenance organization (HMO); and (2) a capitation payment system, in which the physician is paid a predetermined amount for each patient for which she assumes responsibility (rather than each service she renders) during a given period of time. Note that the capitation method can be applied via some type of organization, for example, an HMO; in that case the capitation payment is made to the HMO, which in turn pays the physician in the manner decided by the HMO.

fee schedule   A list of charges (or allowances) for specific procedures and services.

FEHBP   See *Federal Employee Health Benefit Program.*

FEP   See *Federal Employee Health Benefit Program.*

fiduciary   A person who has a legal duty, created by his or her undertaking, to act primarily for the benefit of another or others in matters connected with the undertaking. The fiduciary owes a higher duty of care than a person acting only for his or her own benefit. Guardians, trustees, directors, and executors are traditional fiduciaries. Also, as managed care takes hold, and an intermediary (managed care plan or insurance company, for instance) makes decisions concerning an individual's access to medical care, it is becoming clear that the intermediary is a fiduciary and must act in the best interests of the patient. It must be noted that courts have traditionally been very protective of those to whom a fiduciary duty is owed, so a "breach" of that duty can have very serious consequences.

"Fiduciary" is also used as an adjective, to describe the duty of a fiduciary: a trustee has a fiduciary duty to protect the assets of the hospital.

field   See *data element.*

Financial Accounting Standards Board (FASB)   A professional group which establishes standards for record-keeping, performance, reporting, and ethics for the accounting profession.

financial director   See *chief financial officer (CFO).*

financial statement   A "picture" of the financial condition of an institution, which consists of a "balance sheet" and an "income and expense statement."

financial structure   The portion of an organization's balance sheet which shows how its assets are financed.

financing (finance)   A method of obtaining money. Types available to hospitals include debt financing (borrowing money), equity financing (selling ownership—shares of stock—in the institution), tax-exempt bond financing (if available), and obtaining donations (of decreasing prominence at present).

debt financing   Obtaining money by borrowing.

equity financing   Obtaining money by selling ownership in the organization (usually shares of stock).

tax-exempt bond financing   The sale of tax-exempt bonds (see *bond*) in order to raise money.   In some instances, nonprofit hospitals (see *hospital*) are permitted to issue tax-exempt bonds (a privilege ordinarily held only by government entities) and thus may use this form of financing.

financing (health care)   A method of paying for health care ("health care financing").

finding   An item of information about a patient which can only be elicited by laboratory, X-ray, or other diagnostic procedure, or by observation of the patient's response to therapy.   The physician relies on signs (disturbances of appearance or function which can be detected by the physician or another observer), symptoms (disturbances of appearance, function, or sensation of which the patient is or should be aware), and findings in making a diagnosis.

firewall   A defensive security system consisting of either, or both, hardware and software designed to protect computers from unwanted outside electronic intrusion, rather than direct physical tampering or theft.   The term has gained significance as more and more computers are connected to each other via electronic networks, such as the Internet, where such unwanted electronic intrusion is now possible.   A computer that is never physically connected to an outside network would not typically need a firewall.

first-dollar coverage   See *first-dollar coverage* under *insurance coverage*.

fiscal   Having to do with finance.

fiscal function   The sum of the activities, wherever performed, through which the hospital achieves fiscal (financial) soundness.

fiscal intermediary   An agency, usually a Blue Cross Plan or private insurance company, selected by health care providers to pay claims under Medicare.   Sometimes referred to simply as "intermediary."

fiscal period   An accounting period.   A fiscal period is usually a year, and is therefore called a fiscal year (FY).

fiscal year (FY)   An accounting period which covers exactly one year, at the end of which books are closed, and the year's financial situation summarized.   The fiscal year may or may not be the calendar year.

501(c)(*)   Section 501(section)(numbered paragraph) of the United States Internal Revenue Code of 1954 (as subsequently amended).   Section 501(c) is the section dealing with nonprofit organizations exempt from federal income taxes.   Any organization, to qualify for tax-exempt status under the Internal Revenue Code, must be incorporated in a given state as a nonprofit organization.   Such incorporation, of itself, is not sufficient to grant exemption from federal income taxes.   This exemption is granted only if the IRS, following application by the organization, makes a "determination" that the organization is properly qualified under a specific paragraph.   Each numbered paragraph deals with a "class" of such qualified nonprofit organizations. For example, "501(c)(1) organizations" are those exempt from income taxes because they have been organized under Acts of Congress; "501(c)(16)" organizations are those organized to finance crop operations.

Three classes of organizations in health care find the 501(c)(*) classification of particular interest at this time for two primary reasons: (1) relief from income taxes gives all of them a substantial savings, and (2) for those qualifying for 501(c)(3) classification ("501(c)(3) organizations"), the ability to obtain tax-deductible contributions from foundations and individuals may provide significant income. The three classifications are:

501(c)(3)   The classification reserved for nonprofit organizations which are one or more of the following: primarily those that are charitable, scientific, religious, or educational. Nonprofit hospitals fall into this category, as do churches, and educational institutions. 501(c)(3) organizations are able to obtain tax-deductible donations from individuals and grants from foundations (foundations ordinarily are not able to make grants to organizations, even though the organizations are nonprofit, unless the grantee has obtained this designation from the IRS). Foundations routinely request evidence that the applicant has obtained the 501(c)(3) determination from the IRS.

501(c)(4)   The classification for nonprofit organizations which, while they may be similar to hospitals in many respects, do not satisfy the IRS that they are charitable. HMOs and PHOs typically are given this classification. They are then exempt from paying federal income taxes (this results in a substantial reduction in their operating costs), but contributions to them are not tax-deductible to the donor. Thus they are ineligible for grants from foundations and tax-deductible gifts from individuals.

501(c)(6)   The classification typically described as that for nonprofit "trade associations." State and national professional associations, such as those of physicians, and associations of organizations, such as hospitals, usually qualify for this classification.

501(c)(3) corporation   A nonprofit organization which has been granted a "determination" by the Internal Revenue Service (IRS) that it meets the requirements under Section 501(c)(3) of the *Internal Revenue Code* for classification as "scientific, educational, religious, or charitable," and thus is exempt from federal income taxes, and may receive donations which are "tax-deductible" to the donating individual, foundation, or corporation. Such status is often required by organizations which give grants.

flexible spending account (FSA)   An account managed by an employer that allows employees to set aside pretax funds for medical, dental, legal, and day-care services. FSAs may be components of "cafeteria plans" for providing health care which allow employees to choose among various levels of benefits.

focus group   A group of individuals convened to give their thoughts on a given subject. Focus groups are being used, for example, in market research.

Food and Drug Administration (FDA)   The agency of the federal government responsible for controlling the sale and use of drugs, including the licensing of new drugs for use in humans.

for-profit An entity organized under any of various business forms (corporation, partnership, sole-proprietorship, etc.) whose profits (excess of income over expenses) are returned to its members (shareholders, investors, owners) as dividends. See *for-profit corporation* under *corporation*, and *for-profit hospital* under *hospital*. Distinguished from *nonprofit*, which see.

formulary A document containing recipes for the preparation (compounding) of medicinal drugs. An example of such a volume is the National Formulary (NF), an official publication of the United States Pharmacopeia Convention (USPC). Pharmacopeias, issued by various nations, contain not only the recipes, but also standards as to the strengths and purity of drugs (see *pharmacopeia*). In the United States, USPC also issues the Pharmacopeia of the United States of America (USP), which is a legal standard.

A health care plan (or insurer) may have a "formulary" which is a list of all drugs which are covered by the plan. Within the hospital, the term formulary is applied to the list of drugs which are routinely stocked by the hospital pharmacy and which are available for immediate dispensing; drugs not in the formulary will have to be obtained by special order from other sources.

fourth party A term sometimes used in health care financing. The first two parties are the patient and the provider. The third party is a payer other than the patient, such as Blue Cross and Blue Shield (BC/BS), commercial insurance, or government. The term "fourth party" is sometimes used to designate industry or business, which buys health care for its employees, with or without the services of a third party.

fraud Obtaining products, services, or reimbursement by intentional false statements. Fraud includes such acts as misrepresenting eligibility or need for services, and claiming reimbursement for services not rendered or for nonexistent patients. Fraud is illegal and may carry civil and criminal penalties. Medicare law specifically prohibits fraud; see *fraud and abuse*.

fraud and abuse The criminal misuse of the Medicare system. The crime consists of such behavior as filing false claims for Medicare reimbursement (such as for nonexistent patients, or services that were never performed), paying or receiving "kickbacks" for patient referral, and so forth. Fraud and abuse is a felony which may be punished by fines up to $25,000 or five years in prison, or both, and automatic suspension from participation in Medicare and Medicaid.

free-standing facility A facility which is not a physical part of a hospital or other health care facility. A free-standing facility may be a facility for carrying out ambulatory surgery, urgent care, emergency care, or other care. "Free-standing" does not necessarily indicate separate ownership; a hospital may operate a free-standing facility or the facility may be owned by a separate organization.

freedom-of-choice A policy which permits patients to choose their own physicians. Such choice is at least restricted for persons who are members of an HMO or other managed care plan, because they must go to physicians within the plan (or themselves pay for care obtained elsewhere). In some HMOs patients must be satisfied with the physician on call.

freedom-of-choice waiver   A waiver which excuses the purchaser of care from permitting freedom of choice to the beneficiaries. Freedom of choice is a normal requirement for Medicaid; a state, for example, wishing to carry out its Medicaid plan via managed care would need such a waiver.

FSA   See *flexible spending account.*

FTC   See *Federal Trade Commission.*

FTE   See *full-time equivalent.*

full-time equivalent (FTE)   A concept used in developing statistics on the size of a work force. The idea is to express a work force made up of both full- and part-time employees as the number of workers that would be employed if all were full time. It is computed by dividing the total hours worked by all employees in a given time period by the number of work hours in the time period. Thus an FTE would be, for example, one person working a normal work week, two people working half time, and so on.

fund (verb)   To set aside an asset for a specific purpose, e.g., to "fund depreciation" means to set aside money at a rate determined by estimating the time before a given piece of equipment will have to be replaced so that, at the end of that time, there will be enough money to replace it.

fund (noun)   An asset set aside for a given purpose, e.g., a building fund, which is to be used only for that purpose.

bond sinking fund   A fund in which assets are accumulated in order to liquidate bonds at or before their maturity dates.

compensation fund   See *alternative dispute resolution (ADR).*

debt service fund   See *debt service reserve fund (DSRF).*

debt service reserve fund (DSRF)   A fund to account for accumulating and paying out the funds necessary to retire long term debt which is not to be paid from specific sources. The term is used especially in government accounting. Synonym(s): debt service fund.

endowment fund   A fund whose principal must be kept intact; only the interest income from the fund may be used. Sometimes called a permanent fund.

general fund   Money that can be used; that is, money that has not been set aside ("funded") for a specific purpose. In governmental usage, the "general fund" has the same meaning, that is, it has not been set aside for social security, for example. Synonym(s): unrestricted fund.

permanent fund   See *endowment fund.*

sinking fund   Usually refers to a fund in which money is set aside to pay off financial obligations, for example, to retire bonds.

specific-purpose fund A fund the principal and interest from which can only be used for the purpose specified. The restriction may be imposed by the terms of a gift or by governing body action.

unrestricted fund See *general fund.*

fund balance A term often used by nonprofit organizations in their financial statements to indicate the difference between assets and liabilities. A positive fund balance is sometimes called a gain; in the profit sector, it would be called a profit. A negative fund balance is a loss in either sector. Nonprofit organizations may also refer to the fund balance as "revenues over (under) expenses."

fund-raising Planned and coordinated activities by which the organization seeks gifts. Fund-raising goes under the term "development," and the fund-raising director is called "the director of development."

funds Available money resources. A number of kinds of funds are discussed in connection with hospital finance:

board-designated funds Funds which were unrestricted funds but were later set aside by action of the governing body for specific purposes or projects.

restricted funds Funds that can be expended only for the specific purpose for which they were obtained.

unrestricted funds Funds which the governing body can use at its discretion, as contrasted with restricted funds, those which can only be used for the purpose for which they were given or obtained.

futile care Useless; vain. Treatment, other than comfort care, which will not result in improvement or cure and which could not, in the opinion of the physician (and, usually, consultants), reasonably be expected to result in a quality of life which would be acceptable to the patient.

futility policy A hospital policy dealing with the issues presented by futile care.

FY See *fiscal year.*

G

gainsharing Sharing with employees any increase in revenue which is the result of gains in productivity. Gainsharing is a form of incentive program or profit-sharing (the term "profit" is not used in the nonprofit environment).

gaming Attempting to manipulate "the system" in an illegal or unethical manner. The terms "gaming" and "to game the system" are used, for example, in connection with efforts to bill under the prospective payment system (PPS) in such a way as to maximize income by giving as the principal diagnosis (see *diagnosis*) that diagnosis which places the patient in the highest-priced Diagnosis Related Group (DRG), even though a lower-priced one more correctly reflects the patient's problem and the services rendered.

GAO   See *General Accounting Office.*

gatekeeper   The person responsible for determining the services to be provided to a patient and coordinating the provision of the appropriate care. The purposes of the gatekeeper's function are: (1) to improve the quality of care by considering the whole patient, that is, all the patient's problems and other relevant factors; (2) to ensure that all necessary care is obtained; and (3) to reduce unnecessary care (and cost). When, as is often the case, the gatekeeper is a physician, she or he is a primary care physician and usually must, except in an emergency, give the first level of care to the patient before the patient is permitted to be seen by a secondary care physician. In fact, the gatekeeper must refer the patient for the secondary care. It has been suggested that the term "primary care manager (PCM)" replace the widely-used term "gatekeeper," but "gatekeeper" is likely to be retained.

gatekeeper mechanism   See *gatekeeper.*

gateway   In computer networking terms, any method by which a user can access the resources of one online network while being connected to another. A subscriber of CompuServe, for instance, may also access resources on the *Internet*, or MEDLINE, while maintaining an account and connection only with CompuServe. Gateways can simplify life for the user because there is only a single entry point that needs to be learned and maintained, yet access to resources is limited only by the number of gateways the service provider makes available.

GDP   See *gross domestic product.*

General Accounting Office (GAO)   The agency of the federal government which is the auditing arm of the legislative branch and its financial consultant.

General Health Policy Model (GHPM)   See *well-year.*

generic   Relating to or characteristic of a whole group. The term is often used in connection with drugs, where the meaning is slightly different; in this usage, a drug is "generic" when it is dispensed under its chemical name rather than under the proprietary or trade name of a particular firm's brand of that chemical. When a drug is initially introduced it typically has been patented, and cannot be manufactured by other firms except under license or until expiration of the patent. When the patent expires, however, other firms may produce the drug under their own trade names. When the patent protection has been removed, the drug may be sold as a generic equivalent (under its chemical name), usually at a lower price than under a brand name.

   "Generic" is also used in this volume to describe a term which applies to a class of things, of which there are several types, each of which would be a specific rather than a generic type. For example, the term "steering committee" is described as "generic," while the term "building program steering committee" would be "specific."

generic equivalent (drug)   A drug sold under its chemical (generic) name when patent and trademark protection for the drug under a proprietary or trade name has expired. Generic equivalents are generally less costly than the trademarked product. In many states, substitution of a generic equivalent by a pharmacist is permitted (or required) unless the physician specifically orders that the trademarked product be dispensed. The physician who specifically describes a trademarked product may feel that the generic drug has some differences not detectable by simple chemical analysis; for example, he may believe that its ability to dissolve may not be as good as the brand name product, or that it is not produced with as good quality control as that of a major drug firm which he trusts. The physician's reasons for choosing a trademarked product over a generic one are often well-founded.

genuine progress indicator (GPI)   A measure of the national economy which takes into account such factors as depletion of natural resources, the costs of crime, the household and volunteer economy, defensive expenditures (other than against crime), the distribution of income, and the loss of leisure. The GPI is a start toward an economic indicator to replace the gross domestic product (GDP), which is based entirely on money and industrial and service production data and thus does not allow for other factors which bear on the satisfaction of people with the condition of the nation. It is suggested by its authors that such an indicator would be a better guide to public policy than the GDP. The GPI is the product of Redefining Progress, a nonprofit public-policy organization in San Francisco.

geographic practice cost indices (GPCIs)   A method used to adjust payments made to Medicare providers based on their geographical location. Pronounced "gypsies". See *Omnibus Budget Reconciliation Act of 1989*.

German-style system   A regulated multipayer system of health care. In Germany, approximately 1200 nonprofit insurance plans, called *Krankenkasse* or "sickness funds," are organized by employers, labor unions, and professional groups. The plans are funded by equal payroll taxes on both employers and employees. Self-employed and wealthier employees may purchase private insurance. Funds are turned over to regional networks of physicians, who reimburse doctors in private practice, and to hospitals, who pay their staff physicians. Physician networks oversee their members' utilization. The government oversees fee negotiations which set global budgets, and also covers the poor and the unemployed.

GHPM   General Health Policy Model. See discussion under *well-year*.

global budgeting   A limit on total health care spending for a given unit of population, taking into account all sources of funds. In health care reform discussions and proposals, it usually means that caps will be placed on (1) employers' expenditures, based on payroll, (2) individuals' expenditures for insurance, based on income, (3) institutional budgets' "core spending," and (4) personal out-of-pocket expenditures. Problem areas include how the information on total spending data is obtained or how the "cap" is enforced.

global fee   A single fee charged for certain medical services which would otherwise be broken down into a number of separate fees. Managed care plans frequently use this method to achieve greater predictability of costs, since there otherwise could be significant variations in what separate services the provider actually bills for. For any complex surgery, for instance, there are office visits before and after the actual surgery, and a global fee encompasses all of these services in one single fee. See also *unbundling*.

GNP See *gross national product*.

going bare Slang for practicing without professional liability insurance coverage.

good faith A legal term which means honest in fact, and describes the state of mind of someone acting without intent to defraud or injure, but with the intent of carrying out his legal and professional obligations honestly and fairly, without ulterior or dishonest motive.

Good Samaritan statute A state law which protects a volunteer who stops at the scene of an accident and assists the victims, making that volunteer immune from suit as long as he did not act maliciously or recklessly. Most states have such a law.

governing board See *governing body*.

governing body The body which is legally responsible for the hospital's policies, organization, management, and quality of care. It is often called the "hospital board," "board of trustees," "governing board," or "board of directors." Individual members of the body are "trustees" or "directors," depending on the name of the body. The governing body is accountable to the owner of the hospital, which may, for example, be a corporation, a unit of government, or the community (see *accountability*).There is a growing tendency to call the governing body the "board of directors" in order to emphasize its role in establishing policy and directing the hospital toward goals. The term "board of trustees" is losing some favor because trusteeship may be equated with safeguarding rather than achieving. Synonym(s): hospital board, board of trustees, governing board, board of directors.

GPCIs Geographic Practice Cost Indices. Pronounced "gypsies". See complete definition under *Omnibus Budget Reconciliation Act of 1989*.

GPI See *genuine progress indicator (GPI)*.

granny dumping See *granny dumping* under *dumping*.

grant A sum of money given by the government, a foundation, or other organization to support a program, project, organization, or individual.

> **block grant** A type of health grant from the federal government in which a "block" of money is provided, and the recipient is given relatively broad discretion in its use.

> **categorical grant** Federal funds which have been provided for specific purposes; for example, the treatment of cancer or the establishment of a burn center.

gross domestic product (GDP) The market value of all goods and services produced by labor and property *within* the U.S. during a particular period of time. Income from overseas operations of a domestic corporation would not be included in the GDP, but activities carried on within U.S. borders by a foreign company would be. The GDP measures how the U.S. *economy* is doing.

In 1991, the GDP replaced the gross national product (GNP) to bring the U.S. into greater conformity with international measures of national income. See also *national health expenditures (NHE)* and *Genuine Progress Indicator (GPI)*.

gross national product (GNP)   The market value of all goods and services produced by labor and property supplied by residents of the U.S. during a particular period of time. Income from overseas operations of a domestic corporation would be included in the GNP, which measures how U.S. *residents* are doing economically. See *gross domestic product (GDP)*.

group practice   See *practice (business)*.

group purchasing   See *purchasing*.

GROUPER   A specific computer program (logic) by which patient bills under Medicare are classified to their Diagnosis Related Groups (DRGs), using the Uniform Hospital Discharge Data Set (UHDDS) which contains up to five diagnoses and four procedures (see *diagnosis* and *procedure*) coded by the International Classification of Diseases, 9th Revision, Clinical Modification (ICD-9-CM) along with other standardized information about the patient.

guaranty fund   A pool of money, funded by assessing insurers, which is designed to protect health care providers and consumers if an insurer becomes insolvent.

guest bed program   See *hotel-hospital*.

Guide to the Health Care Field (AHA Guide)   An annual directory of hospitals, multihospital systems, health-related organizations, and American Hospital Association (AHA) members, published by AHA.

guidelines   Directing principles which lay out a suggested policy or procedure.

administrative guidelines   Suggestions promulgated by an administrative agency as to procedure or interpretations of law. Guidelines are not binding as are regulations, which have the force of law. However, they are strongly influential.

clinical practice guidelines   Statements by authoritative bodies as to the procedures appropriate for a physician to employ for certain diagnoses, conditions, or situations. They are intended to change providers' practice styles, reduce inappropriate and unnecessary care, and cut costs. The first guidelines were for the management of a given diagnosis or of the treatment planned. More recently, other topics pertaining to health have appeared, for example, "Driving Following a Single Seizure."

The Agency for Health Care Policy and Research (AHCPR) has been charged with responsibility for producing "Clinical Practice Guidelines (CPGs)," and has issued a number of them. Several medical associations and specialty societies, as well as hospitals, have also published guidelines for various kinds of patients. At least 2,000 guidelines are now in print, although a recent issue of the AMA publication *Practice Parameters Update*, which listed about 100 newly published parameters, also listed about 35 parameters which had been withdrawn during the same period. So the number of and titles of those *in force* is constantly changing.

The term "guidelines" has not been well-received by the American Medical

Association (AMA), which prefers "practice parameters," apparently because "guidelines" has been used for governmental pronouncements, which appear more legally binding. An AMA spokesperson has stated, "practice parameters are not like laws; they're published in journals, and it's up to each person to keep current about what's going on."

Guidelines are not the answer to controlling or improving quality, or controlling cost. Guidelines must necessarily be so broad that they will only identify extreme *under-* and *over-*utilization for a given diagnosis or procedure, or disclose conspicuously egregious practice. There is no way they can be tailored to the individual patient. They also raise serious questions with regard to malpractice, just a few of which are: (1) Is it OK to do *everything* in a guideline? (2) *Must* one do everything within a guideline? (3) If one stays within a guideline does this grant immunity from malpractice? (4) What if a guideline is withdrawn (as about one-third of them are) and a physician still follows it? For potentially better solutions, see *critical path* and *problem-knowledge coupler.*

Also called "practice guidelines, practice parameters, guidelines for medical care."

Health Planning Guidelines   A set of guidelines, issued by the United States Department of Health and Human Services (DHHS) in response to 1974 federal legislation, to assist state and local health planning agencies with their activities and policies.

H

HA   See *health alliance (HA).*

HAD   See *health care alternatives development.*

hardware   The physical components of the computer (keyboard, cathode ray tube, disk drives, and so on), as contrasted with the computer programs, which are called "software." Synonym(s): computer hardware.

Hawaii plan   The health care reform plan instituted in Hawaii in 1974 with passage of a law which required all employers to provide health insurance for all employees working 20 hours a week or more. For the indigent and Medicaid, the insurance is subsidized by the government. Over 95% of Hawaiians are covered by health insurance vs. about 85% on the mainland. Hawaiians claim "near-universal" coverage. The Hawaii plan is advanced by some as a model for the entire U.S., citing Hawaii's lower spending for health care (9% vs. 13% for the U.S. as a whole, despite a higher cost of living in Hawaii) and its statistical evidence, such as lower rates of hospitalization and lower death rates for certain conditions. Critics insist that we must lower our costs before we can provide as extensive coverage and achieve better health, while Hawaiian advocates claim that the greater coverage in Hawaii provides preventive care which is the cause of the lower costs. Critics also fault Hawaii for the uninsured population which still exists there, and the "makeshift" efforts to close the gap. Hawaii is held up as a model of the successful financing of health care by *employer mandate* (sometimes referred to as "pay or play"). See *mandate*.

hazardous materials Substances, such as radioactive or chemical materials, which are dangerous to humans and other living things. Many hospitals have "hazardous materials plans" which are similar to (and sometimes incorporated within) their disaster preparedness plans and which deal specifically with handling emergencies involving hazardous materials. In the event of a nuclear or toxic chemical accident, the plan would go into effect.

For example, a special entrance to the hospital is required to permit control over incoming patients, so that they and their clothing may be decontaminated; hospital staff must be specially garmented; air flow must be controlled to prevent contamination of other areas of the hospital; and so on.

hazardous waste Waste materials which are dangerous to living things, and so require special precautions for disposal. Hazardous waste includes radioactive materials, toxic chemicals, and biological waste (blood, tissue, etc.) which can transmit disease (also called "infectious waste"). In health care, items disposed of regularly include used hypodermic needles, surgical sponges, and other products containing blood and body fluids. A special concern is contaminated needles; a needlestick is one way in which AIDS and hepatitis B can be transmitted. Hospitals are taking great care to ensure proper disposal of hazardous waste; precautions include special, stick-proof containers for needles, colored bags to signal biological waste (red, for example), and other special handling.

HCBSP See *Hospital Community Benefits Standards Program*.

HCCA See *health care coverage area*.

HCFA See *Health Care Financing Administration*.

HCI See *Health Commons Institute*.

HCO See *health care organization*.

HCPCS See *Health Care Financing Administration Common Procedure Coding System*.

HCPOTP Health care professionals other than physicians.

HCPR Health Care Policy and Research. See *Agency for Health Care Policy and Research (AHCPR)*.

health As defined by the World Health Organization (WHO), "the extent to which an individual or group is able, on the one hand, to develop aspirations and satisfy needs; and, on the other hand, to change or cope with the environment. Health is therefore seen as a resource for everyday life, not the objective of living; it is seen as a positive concept emphasizing social and personal resources, as well as physical capacities." In common usage, "health" often is used to refer to the condition of physical, mental, and social well-being, and is much like the word "quality" in that it is modified by adjectives in such phrases as "poor health," "good health," or "failing health." It is worth noting that increasing attention is being given to quality of life.

health advocacy An allied health field which originated as "patient advocacy," that is, efforts to help resolve patients' complaints in relation to medical care and hospital and other health care services and with the protection of their rights. Thus health advocacy was originally the field of the patient advocate or patient representative, also known as an "ombudsperson."

Today, however, the person who serves as the advocate of an individual patient's interests is but one variety of "health advocate." Health advocacy is practiced not only by patient advocates, but also by advocates for groups of people in health programs, by program specialists in health foundations, by patient advocates for special populations or interest groups, and by legislative specialists in health. The current trend is for this broader advocacy to be a joint effort of consumers and professionals.

health advocate See *patient advocate*.

health alliance (HA) An organization which was proposed in the health care reform legislation to be established in the managed competition approach to health care reform to serve as a "sponsor" for populations which would otherwise have no intermediary between their beneficiaries and organizations which provide care. Its basic functions are to bargain with and purchase health insurance from accountable health plans (AHPs) or other sources of health care in behalf of consumers, and to furnish information to consumers on the services provided by the competing AHPs, an evaluation of their quality of care, participant satisfaction, and price.

Health alliances are not needed for groups such as corporations with many employees, state governments, and similar institutions which are large enough effectively to carry out the purchasing function themselves.

When proposed initially, the organization was called a "health insurance purchasing corporation (HIPC)." This was then changed to "health insurance purchasing cooperative (HIPC)" and, later, "health plan purchasing cooperative (HPPC)." All were referred to as "hippick", an acronym no one could look up in a glossary. Another recent synonym is "insurance purchasing pool." The current terminology seems to be settling to "health alliance."

health care Services of health care professionals and their agents which are addressed at: (1) health promotion; (2) prevention of illness and injury; (3) monitoring of health; (4) maintenance of health; and (5) treatment of diseases, disorders, and injuries in order to obtain cure or, failing that, optimum comfort and function (quality of life).

health care alternatives development (HAD) A term that refers to the development of alternative delivery systems and alternative financing systems. One must seek the context of this term to understand just what is meant.

health care coalition An organization working on broad health care concerns, ordinarily including hospital and health care costs, and typically with provider, business, and consumer participation. Often there is government participation as well.

business health care coalition   A health care coalition comprised of or organized by business firms concerned with health care problems, primarily those problems affecting employees of the member companies. Such a coalition is also likely to have providers and consumers as members.

health care consultant   A person who holds herself or himself out as an independent contractor to provide professional advice and services to hospitals, often concerning management matters and planning. The American Association of Healthcare Consultants (AAHC) recognizes consultants in several specialties: Strategic Planning and Marketing; Organization and Management; Human Resource Management; Facilities Programming and Planning; Finance; Operations and Information Systems; and Health Specialist. Synonym(s): hospital consultant.

health care delivery   A term sometimes used as a synonym for "comprehensive health care delivery system." However, the term "health care delivery" applies to providing any of the wide array of health care services as well as to the totality.

health care delivery system   A term without specific definition, referring to all the facilities and services, along with methods for financing them, through which health care is provided.

Health Care Financing Administration (HCFA)   The division of the Department of Health and Human Services (DHHS) which administers the Medicare and Medicaid programs at the federal level.

Health Care Financing Administration Common Procedure Coding System (HCPCS)   A federal coding system used to identify medical services and supplies provided to Medicare patients. Pronounced "hick-picks", this coding system includes the *Physicians' Current Procedural Terminology (CPT)* codes copyrighted by the American Medical Association, as well as additional codes to include services and supplies not covered by the CPT codes. While all CPT codes are numeric only (five digits), HCPCS use the format of one letter followed by four digits. Letters A-V are reserved for nation-wide use, while letters W-Z are available to local Medicare carriers. Some alphanumeric code examples are A0010 for an ambulance ride, A4927 for gloves, A9300 for exercise equipment, D7130 for a tooth root removal, G0008 for a flu shot ("Admin influenza virus vac") , P9610 for collecting a urine specimen, and V2020 for a pair of glasses (no kidding!).

health care institution   As commonly used, any institution dealing with health. Some definitions state that an institution, to qualify for this term, must have an organized professional staff. However, there are no regulations, such as standards for the licensure or registry of institutions, which currently restrict the use of this term.

health care organization (HCO)   An organizational form for health care delivery in which the financial risk (health care) is assumed by the organization, rather than by individuals.

health care plan An organized service to provide stipulated medical, hospital, and related services (benefits) to individuals under a prepayment contract. The plan may be offered by a Blue Cross/Blue Shield (BC/BS) plan, an insurance company, a health maintenance organization (HMO), a health care organization (HCO), or other organization.

Health Care Policy and Research See *Agency for Health Care Policy and Research (AHCPR)*.

Health Care Prepayment Plan (HCPP) A prepaid plan serving Medicare beneficiaries based on reimbursement, not risk. The Health Care Financing Administration (HCFA) will provide reimbursement for services actually provided. Distinguished from HMOs and similar plans in that HCPPs do not need to provide all Medicare covered services, do not have to offer open enrollment, and can avoid member appeal rights. HCPPs are frequently used by labor organizations to provide services for their members only.

health care professional See *health care professional* under *professional*.

health care proxy See *advance directive*.

health care reform A term without a clear definition, which is applied to the efforts on the federal, state, and local levels to make changes in the health care delivery "system" so that (1) costs are reduced or "contained," (2) the uninsured population, estimated at 35-40 million people nationally, are covered; (3) all citizens have access to health care, (4) financing is assured, and (5) quality of care is controlled or, preferably, improved. The options as to "management" of the health care system range from highly centralized, federal controls, through the setting of certain requirements at the federal or state level but allowing local innovation as to implementation, through local solutions even if nothing is done at the state or national level.

health care system A system designed to take responsibility only for the *care* of those who seek it out. It responds to the needs of individual patients who present themselves with illness or injury. See *health system*.

Health Commons Institute (HCI) A nonprofit corporation dedicated to applying modern information technology at the person-health care system clinical interface. The primary such interface is the patient-physician encounter and relationship. The name of the organization was derived from the concept of a "commons" as a meeting ground.

HCI was established in 1992 as a result of the beliefs of its founders and others that the potential now exists for a true paradigm shift in health care, characterized in part by a change in the locus of control of health care and decision making from doctors toward patients and their families. Trends supporting this belief include: (1) today's Americans increasingly want to make their own choices in matters of health and health care; (2) wise choices can only be made where complete, but patient- and problem- specific, information is available and intelligible at the place and time of decision making; (3) only through modern information technology (i.e., the computer) is it possible to meet this information requirement, because the volume of biomedical literature is overwhelming (see *Problem-Knowledge Coupler* as an example of an approach to this problem); and (4) "patients" often need the help of the health care professional in the analysis of their problems, in interpretation of the biomedical information, and in making choices among their options as to health promotion, disease prevention, health problem solution, and therapy.

HCI's mission is to study and facilitate this paradigm shift with respect to: physician (and other professional) education; patient education; public education; health care practice design; health care cost; effects on personal health; community health outcomes achieved; public health practice; legal implications for information technology, licensure, and malpractice considerations; computer hardware and software application and development; library and other information management; medical record systems.

health economics The branch of economics (a social science) which deals with the provision of health care services, their delivery, and their use, with special attention to quantifying the demands for such services, the costs of such services and of their delivery, and the benefits obtained. More emphasis is given to the costs and benefits of health care to a population than to the individual.

health education See *education.*

health facility licensing agency A state agency which sets standards and issues permits for the operation of health facilities.

health fair A type of community health education activity in which exhibits are the main method used and in which free diagnostic services such as chest X-rays and multiphasic screening are sometimes offered.

health hazard appraisal (HHA) See *health risk appraisal.*

Health Insurance Association of America (HIAA) An organization made up of companies writing health insurance.

Health Insurance for the Aged See *Medicare.*

health insurance purchasing cooperative (HIPC) See *health alliance.*

health IRA See *individual health care account.*

health maintenance All efforts carried out in order to preserve health. As used in the term health maintenance organization (HMO), however, the term is not so inclusive, but rather simply includes those health care services which are included in the particular benefit package of the enrollee.

health maintenance organization (HMO) A health care providing organization which ordinarily has a closed group ("panel") of physicians (and sometimes other health care professionals), along with either its own hospital or allocated beds in one or more hospitals. Individuals (usually families) "join" an HMO, which agrees to provide "all" the medical and hospital care they need, for a fixed, predetermined fee. Actually, each subscriber is under a contract stipulating the limits of the service (not "all" the care needed). Such a contract is called a risk contract and the HMO is therefore called a "risk contractor."

open-ended health maintenance organization (open-ended HMO)   See *point-of-service plan (POS)*.

social/health maintenance organization (S/HMO)   A newer type of long-term care (LTC) "alternative" organization under experimentation in which one provider, under a capitation payment (a fixed fee for each individual covered), furnishes both social and health care services for (currently) low income individuals.

health plan purchasing cooperative (HPPC)   See *health alliance* .

health planning   See *health planning* under *planning*.

health planning guidelines   See *Health Planning Guidelines* under *guidelines*.

health professional shortage area   An area so designated by the Secretary of Health and Human Services (HHS) under the Public Health Service Act.

health promotion   Efforts to change peoples' behavior in order to promote healthy lives and, to the extent possible, prevent illnesses and accidents and to minimize their effects, rather than having people use the health care system for "repairs." A health promotion program may include health risk appraisal of the individuals, and may give attention to fitness, stress management, smoking, cholesterol reduction, weight control, nutrition, cancer screening, and other matters on the basis of the risks detected. Synonym(s): wellness program.

health-related care institution   A facility providing some kind of health care to inpatients who do not require full nursing services.

health-related services   A term apparently used to include everything in the health care field except medical care (physician services).

health resources   Personnel (both professional and supportive), facilities, funds, and technology which are available or could be made available for health services.

health risk appraisal   A technique for determining for a given individual the factors most likely to result in illness, injury, or premature death. The determination is based on comparing a set of data about the individual (her database) with statistics on the likelihood of specific illnesses, injuries, and causes of death among large groups of persons for whom the same database has been collected and analyzed. Included in the database are the individual's age, sex, physical condition, genetic background, behavior, environment, and other factors, obtained by examination of the individual, laboratory tests, and information obtained from the person by interview or questionnaire.

The purpose of the appraisal is preventive, that is, to be able to prescribe measures and programs to counter the risks detected. For example, elevated blood pressure would be a risk whenever it occurs; inability to swim would be an especially great risk factor in a child exposed to water sports; and driving a motor vehicle would be a risk factor when a patient requires certain drugs which interfere with the ability to drive. Synonym(s): health risk assessment.

health risk assessment   See *health risk appraisal*.

Health Security Act (HSA)   President Clinton's proposal for health care reform, which was defeated in 1993.

health service area   A specific geographic area considered in the governmental health planning process.   The boundaries of health service areas were established in compliance with 1974 federal legislation on the basis of population, political subdivisions, geography, and other factors.   The term "health service area" may also be used more loosely to mean service area, the area from which a facility or program actually draws its patients or clients, that is, its "catchment area."

health services   A term without specific definition which pertains to any services which are health-related.

health services research   Research pertaining to the efficiency and effectiveness of various organizational forms for health care delivery, administrative approaches, relationship to needs, and like matters.

health status   The state of health of an individual or population.   A description of health status is usually given either in vague lay terms, for example, "good," or as a health status index, which may appear more objective and meaningful than it really is.

health status index   A statistic which attempts to quantify the health status of an individual or a population.   Such indices are developed using health status indicators.   Statements of health status have not been developed to the point that they have standard definitions; each publication using such indices should give full details on the indicators used, their aggregation into the indices themselves, and any other pertinent methodological detail, such as the sampling techniques used (in the case of health status indices for populations).

health status indicator   A measurement of some attribute of individual or community health which is considered to reflect health status.   Each attribute is given a numerical value, and a score (a health status index) is calculated for the individual or community from the aggregate of these values.   To the extent possible, the indicators are objective, that is, they are facts for which various observers or investigators would each find the same value.   In the case of a community, such statistics as mortality and morbidity rates are sometimes used.   For health status of individuals (and thus of the group), data may be obtained by sampling (obtaining data on only a properly-selected portion of the population).   Such facts may be obtained by examination of individuals or by questionnaires inquiring as to physical function, quality of life, activities of daily living (ADL), emotional well-being, episodes of medical care, and the like.   Much study has been and is being given to developing indicators and indices of health status.   No standard measures have appeared.   Published data on health status should be "taken with a grain of salt" unless the reader can satisfy herself as to the methodological detail of obtaining data on the indicators and calculating the indices.

health survey   An investigation of an area or population in order to obtain information about some aspect of the health of its population (its health problems, its health resources, or anything else pertaining to health). Such a survey typically employs sampling, and may obtain information from direct observations, questionnaires, published data, or other sources.

health system   A system designed to take responsibility for the *health* of its defined community; it involves "outreach" rather than "response" or "reaction." This is in contrast with a health *care* system (see *health care system*).

health systems agency (HSA)   A nonprofit organization or agency set up under federal law to perform health planning functions, develop a health systems plan, conduct certificate of need (CON) reviews, and review the use of certain federal funds.

health systems plan   A five-year plan prepared by a health systems agency (HSA).

Health Technology Assessment Reports (HTAR)   See *Office of Health Technology Assessment (OHTA)*.

healthy communities movement   A movement which contends that the goal of the health care system should be the health of the community, and that every community is responsible for its own health, that is, for having its own "health system" — of which traditional health care is only a part. To that end, there must be wide involvement of all agencies, organizations, and citizens, and the hospital must fit into the total scheme for achievement of optimum health of the citizens, even though this will alter its traditional role of simply providing care to those who present themselves to it.

healthy community   An unofficial label which a community often gives itself when it has established and continues an organized effort to achieve optimum health for all its residents and visitors, using the resources available, and in response to it's own perceived needs. Such a community is part of the healthy communities movement.

A healthy community finds that it has human resources which can be tapped and mobilized in new and novel ways and financial resources which can be pooled. Organizations and agencies which often have provided duplicate services and competed with one another become collaborators. Services are taken to where the needs are. Physicians, other health care professionals, and hospitals increase their outreach programs.

Among the projects reported in healthy communities are:
> Prenatal care
> Environmental monitoring
> Fitness
> Women's health
> Indigent care
> Migrant workers
> Preventive medicine
> Elder day care
> Injury prevention
> Firearm safety

Companionship for shut-ins
Dental services to children
Water safety instruction
Housing for the homeless
Community-knowledge based managed care
Time Dollars earnings for volunteer services
Parish nursing
Voice mail triage into health care
Teenage pregnancy programs
Consumer health education
School health
Immunization
Consumer health informatics
Voice mail guidance to prenatal care
Domestic violence prevention
"One-stop shopping" for community services
Child abuse prevention
Safety education
Community health information networks
"One-stop shopping" for health care

heroic treatment   See *extraordinary treatment* under *treatment.*

heterogeneous   Composed of a mixture of things. For example, a Diagnosis Related Group (DRG) which is heterogeneous is one that is composed of patients with a variety of diagnoses, as contrasted with a "homogeneous" or "single-diagnosis" group, in which all the patients have the same diagnosis.

hickfa or hickva   Common pronunciations of the acronym HCFA. See *Health Care Financing Administration.*

hick-picks   Common pronunciation of HCPCS. See *Health Care Financing Administration Common Procedure Coding System (HCPCS).*

hikva   A common pronunciation for the acronym HCFA. See *Health Care Financing Administration.*

Hill-Burton program   A 1946 federal program of financial assistance for the construction and renovation of hospitals and other health care facilities. The intent was to increase the number of hospital beds in poor or under-served areas of the United States. By 1978, when the law expired, 500,000 hospital beds had been built, at a cost of about $13.5 billion. In 1994, it was estimated that the U.S. had a surplus of 300,000 hospital beds. Since hospital beds cost about $40,000 each per year to operate, eliminating these beds could save the U.S. about $12 billion.

hippick   Common pronunciation of HIPC or HPPC, for "health insurance purchasing cooperative (HIPC)" or "health plan purchasing cooperative (HPPC)." See *health alliance (HA).*

holding company   A corporation organized for the purpose of owning the stock of another corporation or corporations; or any company which owns such a large portion of the stock of a corporation that it controls that corporation.

holistic health   A view of health as consisting of the health of the "whole" person—body, mind, and spirit. That view requires the coordinated attention to all three components by the several disciplines involved, and places major responsibility for health on the individual. Synonym, wholistic health.

holistic medicine   A term originally applied to the principle that the whole person should be treated, rather than just the person's disease, disturbance of function, or injury. This principle has always guided the provision of health care of good quality, which stresses the importance of personal responsibility, prevention, exercise, nutrition, rest, moderation, personal habits, and so on. Holistic medicine became the focus of a movement in the 1960s with the formation of the International Association of Holistic Health Practitioners (IAHHP) in 1970. The term has come under criticism by the medical profession and others in recent years because it has come to include a variety of treatment methods, some of which are incompatible with others, and some of which have scientific proof while others do not. For example, such a mixed bag of concepts as astrology, nutrition, faith healing, graphology, macrobiotics, naturopathy, numerology, acupuncture, psychocalisthenics, self-massage, psychotherapy, and touch encounter have at various times been listed as among the tools of holistic medicine.

home health care   Care at the levels of skilled nursing care and intermediate care (see *nursing care*) provided in the patient's home through an agency which has the resources necessary to provide that care. The care is given under the prescription of a physician by professional nurses (registered nurses (RNs) and licensed practical nurses (LPNs); see *nurse*), and other health care professionals (social workers, physical therapists, and so forth), as appropriate. Services may also include homemaking and personal care services.

Home health care is a growing alternative to skilled nursing facilities and units (SNFs and SNUs) and to intermediate care facilities (ICFs) and units. Also called "in-home care" and "home care." See also *home life care.*

Often home health care is divided into three categories, depending on the intensity:

home life care   Supportive services provided by an agency in order to permit an individual who is able to carry out the activities of daily living (ADL) to remain at home rather than being placed in an institution. The services are given by homemakers and home aides rather than by nurses. One benefit of having such trained assistance in the home is that the worker going into the home is in a position to detect the need for and to obtain nursing services as required. Home life care is distinguished from home health care in that home health care includes nursing services under the direction of a physician rather than simply homemaking care. See also *home health care.*

homeopathy   See *homeopathy* under *medicine.*

homogeneous   Composed of things which are the same, in contrast to "heterogeneous," which refers to a mixture. For example, in a homogeneous or "single-diagnosis" Diagnosis Related Group (DRG), all the patients have the same diagnosis; on the other hand, a heterogeneous DRG is composed of patients with a variety of diagnoses.

hospice program   A program that assists with the physical, emotional, spiritual, psychological, social, financial, and legal needs of the dying patient and her family. The service may be provided in the patient's home or in an institution (or division of an institution) set up for the purpose. Volunteers are integral parts of the staff. Bereavement care for the family is also included.

hospital   The traditional definition of "hospital" is that it is a health care institution which has an organized professional staff and *medical staff*, and inpatient facilities, and which provides medical, nursing, and related services. States have specific definitions for what may be called a "hospital," including, for example, a minimum number of beds, and the services which must be available.

However, in an increasing number of communities, the term hospital is being applied to a geographic region occupied by a virtual health care organization with multiple programs operating in multiple locations. This emerging hospital is a deinstitutionalized, decentralized, electronically integrated community health care network, which includes churches, schools, neighborhoods, and workplaces. Services are being provided where the people reside and spend their time rather than expecting the people to go to the hospital except for a narrow range of procedural or other services requiring its extraordinary resources.

A given hospital may fit one or more of the following definitions:

accredited hospital   A hospital meeting the standards of the Joint Commission on Accreditation of Healthcare Organizations (JCAHO) and so certified by JCAHO (or, in Canada, by the Canadian Council on Health Facilities Accreditation (CCHFA)).

acute care hospital   A hospital which cares primarily for patients with acute diseases and injuries (that is, those with an average length of stay (ALOS) of 30 days or less), or in which more than half the patients are admitted to units with an ALOS of 30 days or less. Also called an acute hospital and short-term hospital.

affiliated hospital   A hospital that has some connection with another hospital, a training program, a multihospital system, a medical center, or some other organization.

AHA-registered hospital   A hospital recognized by the American Hospital Association (AHA) as meeting its definition of a hospital and approved by its Board of Trustees for registration. Sometimes called simply "registered hospital."

certified hospital   A hospital recognized by the Department of Health and Human Services (DHHS) as meeting the standards necessary to be a provider for Medicare.

chronic disease hospital   See *long-term hospital*.

city hospital   A hospital controlled by a city government. While a hospital operated by a city is often referred to as a "municipal hospital" (and properly can be called that), the term municipal hospital refers to a hospital operated by any municipal government.

community hospital   A hospital established primarily to provide services to the residents of the community in which it is located. Most community hospitals are nonprofit, non-federal, and for short term patients.

community-owned hospital   See *nonprofit hospital*.

county hospital   A hospital controlled by county government.

day care hospital   A hospital which treats, during the day, patients who are able to return to their homes at night.

disproportionate share hospital   A Medicare term for a hospital serving a higher than average proportion of low-income patients.

district hospital   A hospital controlled by a special political subdivision (a "hospital district") created solely to operate the hospital and other health care institutions.

federal government hospital   A hospital controlled and operated by the federal government.

for-profit hospital   A hospital operated by a for-profit corporation, in which the profits are paid in the form of dividends to shareholders who own the corporation. A for-profit hospital is the same as an investor-owned hospital and a proprietary hospital; see also *publicly-owned hospital*.

general hospital   A hospital offering care for a variety of conditions and age groups. It is contrasted with a specialty hospital (for example, a children's hospital, or an "eye and ear" or psychiatric hospital).

government hospital   A hospital which is operated by a unit of government, usually the federal government. Hospitals operated by states are usually called state hospitals, and those operated by cities are usually called municipal hospitals.

investor-owned hospital   See *for-profit hospital*.

licensed hospital   A hospital licensed by the state licensing agency.

long-term hospital   A hospital providing long-term care for patients not in an acute phase of an illness but who require more skilled services than those available in a nursing home. Synonym(s): chronic disease hospital.

municipal hospital   A hospital operated by a municipal government, usually a city.

night hospital   A hospital that treats, only at night, patients who are able to be out during the day.

nondelegated hospital   A hospital not qualified under its Professional Standards Review Organization (PSRO) to perform review functions (see *delegated hospital*).

nonprofit hospital   A hospital owned and operated by a corporation whose "profits" (excess of income over expense) are used for hospital purposes rather than returned to shareholders or investors as dividends. "Nonprofit" does not necessary mean "tax-exempt." To be tax exempt, an organization must not only be nonprofit, but also qualify under paragraph 501(c)(3) of the Internal Revenue Code as "scientific, religious, educational, or charitable" and have a determination to this effect from the IRS. The organization must also meet state requirements to be exempt from state taxes. Synonym(s): community-owned hospital, not-for-profit hospital.

not-for-profit hospital   See *nonprofit hospital.*

private hospital   A hospital not operated by a government agency. A private hospital may be either for-profit or nonprofit.

proprietary hospital   See *for-profit hospital.*

psychiatric hospital   A hospital specializing in the care of patients with mental illness.

publicly-owned hospital   A hospital operated by a corporation which offers ownership of shares to the general public. The term is currently being applied to for-profit, investor-owned (proprietary) hospitals.

registered hospital   Short for AHA-registered hospital.

rehabilitation hospital   A hospital specializing in rehabilitation care.

satellite hospital   A hospital operated by another, "parent," hospital, at a location different than that of the parent hospital.

self-insured hospital   A hospital carrying self-insurance; see *insurance.*

short-term hospital   See *acute care hospital.*

sole community hospital (SCH)   A hospital which is the only reasonably available inpatient facility in a given geographic area, due to the absence of other hospitals, travel time or difficulty, or other reasons.

specialty hospital   A hospital which cares for only a limited category of patients, such as psychiatric, orthopedic, or pediatric patients.

state hospital   A hospital operated by a state. Such hospitals are usually specialized, particularly for the care of contagious disease and psychiatric patients.

teaching hospital   A hospital with one or more accredited education programs in medicine, nursing, or the allied health professions.

university hospital   A hospital which is owned by or affiliated with a medical school and which is used in the education of physicians.

voluntary hospital   A hospital which is private (nongovernmental), autonomous, and self-supported.

hospital chain   See *multihospital system.*

Hospital Community Benefits Standards Program (HCBSP) A voluntary certification program for hospitals, created at New York University by Robert Sigmond and Anthony Kovner, under grant support from the W. K. Kellogg Foundation. The purpose of the program is to stimulate hospitals to provide community benefits, and to reward them with special certification when they do.

The hospital must meet four standards to be certified: (1) the hospital's governing board must define the boundaries of the community and approve the goals and operations plan of the community benefit program, (2) the hospital must sponsor projects that improve the overall health standards in the community, (3) the hospital must identify community health problems and ways to solve them (this effort can be conducted in conjunction with other community organizations and projects), and (4) the hospital must encourage the involvement of a wide range of hospital employees, medical staff members, and volunteers.

hospital consultant See *health care consultant.*

hospital discharge abstract system A system in which a number of hospitals submit coded, computer-ready summaries (discharge abstracts) of clinical records to a central shared computer service. The summaries may be submitted on paper or via computer media. In return, the hospitals receive reports and analyses of their own data, which they need for their internal operations. In addition, by using standardized information, hospitals may obtain interhospital comparisons, and may establish a database which may be used, under the confidentiality rules of the system, for research. The prototype of such systems is the Professional Activity Study (PAS) of the Commission on Professional and Hospital Activities (CPHA).

hospital district A special political subdivision created solely to operate the hospital and other health care institutions.

Hospital Health Plan (HHP) A specific model of physician-hospital organization (PHO) whose managed care plan (MCP) is emerging as an alternative to the typical health maintenance organization (HMO). To the extent that groups and members of the community work with the hospital and physicians in a collaborative effort to create the plan, it is better called a "community health plan." The model was developed by Richard Ya Deau, MD, in 1984. HHPs are established with the assistance of Hospital Health Plan Corporation (HHPC). To use the title Hospital Health Plan (HHP), which is copyrighted by HHPC, a plan must have certain attributes:

(1) An HHP is designed to provide the services needed for its own defined population; it is "community rated" in benefits as well as in premium structure (see *community rating* under *rating*). Its health services are those required for prevention of disease, injury, and disability and for provision of optimal care, with the goal of achieving optimal health for the community rather than simply health care for those who present themselves. It is designed to manage care rather than manage dollars.

(2) An HHP can only be established after a thorough feasibility study and actuarial analysis which provides evidence that the proposed plan will (1) have an adequate enrollment; (2) have adequate participation by providers and others; (3) be able to offer its locally-defined benefit package for a saleable premium; (4) have a sound business and capitalization plan; and (5) be able to meet the state's requirements for licensure as an insurance company (reinsurance protects against

unexpected loss). As a result of this careful preparation, several HHPs are in successful operation (including repaying their start-up financing) with as few as 12-15,000 enrollees.

(3) An HHP is a nonprofit health services organization, and since none of the premium income is committed to shareholders or equity investors, it is able to function with a "medical loss ratio" (portion of the premium spent on benefits) reported to be about 91%. In a nonprofit operation, the higher this ratio is, the better, since the plan exists to provide care. (In a for-profit insurance company, the incentive is to keep this number low (often lower than 75%) in order to reward the investors.) Thus the nonprofit plan can provide more care with a lower premium.

(4) Governance of an HHP is by a local board of directors which includes physicians, health care facilities, and enrollees.

(5) The physicians in the HHP develop the medical policies and oversee their implementation, rather than being overseen by an "outside" HMO.

(6) The hospital(s)' financial survival is insured by including in the financing of the HHP a capitation amount for the predicted hospitalizations for the enrolled population.

(7) Physicians may be paid by either fee-for-service from a capitated pool or directly capitated, depending on the policies of the plan and individual preference.

An HHP has available to it, under license from HHPC, a management information system (MIS) which provides all necessary on-line transactional processing (OLTP) resources for a managed care plan and an on-demand knowledge-based analytic processing system. See discussion of these processing types under *Online Analytical Processing (OLAP)* and *knowledge-based*. This software has been developed for and with a number of operating HHPs, and thus the development and maintenance costs are shared. Each HHP can tailor the software to its own particular needs.

Hospital Health Plan Corporation (HHPC) A corporation in Minnesota which assists communities, their hospitals, and their physicians in establishing Hospital Health Plans (HHPs), and provides startup assistance, continuing support for its transactional and analytical management information system, and liaison with other HHPs.

hospital information system (HIS) See hospital information system (HIS) under *information system*.

Hospital Insurance Program (HI) See *Medicare, Part A*, under *Medicare*.

Hospital Research and Educational Trust (HRET) A nonprofit research arm of the American Hospital Association (AHA), which supports activities to improve hospitals and health services.

Hospital Statistics The annual publication of the American Hospital Association (AHA) covering hospitals in the United States, and giving descriptions of each as well as tabulated data on hospitals.

hospitalization A period of stay in the hospital. Also, the placing of a patient in the hospital.

partial hospitalization Treatment which involves the use of hospital day beds or night beds or adult day care services on a regularly scheduled basis. The services provided may include medical, social, nutritional, psychological, and others.

hotel-hospital   A hotel facility operated by a hospital, at hotel rates, for use by patients and their families before and after hospitalization. Such facilities are sometimes used for temporary care for elderly patients in order to give their family caregivers a rest. If separated from the hospital, the hotel-hospital often provides shuttle bus service. Synonym(s): guest bed program.

hotel, medical care   See *medical care hotel*.

HTAR   Health Technology Assessment Reports. See *Office of Health Technology Assessment (OHTA)*.

I

iatrogenic illness   An illness or injury resulting from a diagnostic procedure, therapy, or other element of health care. An iatrogenic illness is often confused with a "nosocomial" illness, which simply means an illness "occurring in a hospital."

IDN   Integrated delivery network. See *integrated health delivery network (IHDN)*.

IDS   Integrated delivery system. See *integrated health delivery network (IHDN)*.

imaging   A term which covers the variety of technologies which result in pictures (images) of body structures or functioning. The first imaging technology was, perhaps, medical illustration. Then came conventional radiology (X-ray). The next technology to gain prominence was computed tomography (CT) scanning. To these have been added magnetic resonance imaging (MRI), diagnostic ultrasound, single photon emission tomography (SPET), and positron emission tomography (PET). Many former Departments of Radiology in hospitals are now called Departments of Imaging.

IMIS   Integrated management information system. See *management information system (MIS)* under *information system*.

impaired   A descriptive term which, when applied to a professional such as a physician, usually encompasses physical handicaps, alcoholism, drug dependence, senility, mental illness, or, sometimes, behavior problems.

implant   To place a substitute organ, tissue, or device in a living body. The difference between implanting and transplanting is that implanting may involve a device (for example, a cardiac pacemaker, or an artificial hip joint, or a capsule of radioactive material) or an organ or tissue, while transplanting involves only organs or tissues. The term implant may also be used as a noun to indicate the organ or tissue implanted.

implicit   "Naturally" a part of, although not specifically stated. See *explicit* for further discussion.

incentive   A reward for desired behavior. In health care, this term is used in regard to rewards to institutions and individuals for decreasing hospital and physician costs, and for encouraging patients to be frugal in demands for health care. See also *disincentive*.

incentive pay plan   A plan for rewarding the performance of individuals in an institution with added compensation. The incentives typically are in the form of annual bonuses or percentage increments above the base salary if specified financial, productivity, or quality performance goals are met, although some institutions use long-term incentives. A 1991 survey found that about two-thirds of the for-profit hospitals and about half the non-profit hospitals, both secular and religious, offer annual incentives. Although these incentives typically apply to top executive personnel, there is a growing trend to offer group incentives, i.e., incentives to the personnel in various organizational units of the institution.

income   Money earned during an accounting period, in contrast with revenue, which is the increase in assets or the decrease in liabilities during the accounting period.

income and expense statement   A standard part of a financial statement in which are shown the revenues, costs, and expenses of the organization for the accounting period. The other part of the financial statement is the balance sheet. Synonym(s): profit and loss statement (P & L), operating statement, income statement.

income statement   See *income and expense statement*.

incremental   An adjective which describes a process which proceeds step-by-step, and each step adds an increment (increase in quantity or value) to the step preceding. The term is being used with a different meaning in health care reform discussions to mean a process of change which happens bit-by-bit rather than all at once; action in contrast with an approach in which substantial health care reform steps would occur simultaneously. A better word might be "additive." Various actions of reform, such as cost controls and tort reform, for example, taken incrementally would be taken separately. Changes made one at a time might be less traumatic, but would extend the whole reform process over a considerable time, all essential changes might never occur, and generally the end result is not likely to be as complete a change as might be desirable. Furthermore, the pieces, when finally in place, may not fit together well.

indemnity   A term being used now by some writers and speakers to mean "the current system" for paying for health care. Actually, the current insurance system has both "service" benefits programs and "indemnity" benefits, each with a specific legal meaning. See *benefits*.

indemnity benefits or insurance   See *benefits*.

indemnity contract   See *indemnity contract* under *contract*.

independent contractor   A person who works for himself and is not controlled by another, as distinguished from an employee. See *employee* for further discussion.

independent physician association (IPA)   Synonym for *individual practice association (IPA)*.

individual practice association (IPA)   A type of health care provider organization composed of physicians, in which the physicians maintain their own practices but agree to furnish services to patients who have signed up for a prepayment plan in which the physician services are supplied by the IPA.   An IPA is not a health maintenance organization (HMO), a health care organization (HCO), or a preferred provider organization (PPO).

independent practitioner   See *independent practitioner* under *practitioner.*

index (numerical)   A number expressing the relative size of a given statistic (number calculated from data) when compared with a reference value for that statistic. It is the result of dividing the given value of the statistic by the reference value.

> **consumer price index (CPI)**   A statistic produced by the U. S. Department of Labor's Bureau of Labor Statistics (BLS) to measure inflation. The CPI compares the price of a market basket of goods and services in specified cities during a certain month against the average price of the same market basket during a base period.
>
> Changes in hospital and medical costs are compared with changes in a specific portion of the CPI called the Consumer Price Index — Medical Care Services (CPI-MSC). It should be understood that such comparisons may be faulty in that the CPI uses in its computation the cost of hospital services to private patients paying *list* prices. Recent evidence suggests that actual price inflation for hospitals (net rather than list) may be about one-half the figure used in the CPI. This is because of the fact that *very few patients pay list prices.* A growing number of organizations paying for care negotiate discounts, and such discounts are said to be increasing in size. Thus hospital price inflation is far less divergent from the overall CPI than usually stated.
>
> The CPI also has a pharmaceutical component, CPI-Rx, which uses retail prices of various types of drugs.
>
> Related to the CPI is the "Producer Price Index — Hospital (PPI-H)", introduced by the BLS in 1993, which measures net changes in hospital prices (as opposed to costs) for a standardized patient against a baseline using the same computation for December 1992. Thus the CPI-MSC and the PPI-H are measuring different aspects of health care costs or prices.

> **economic index**   A statistical measure of the economy. One such index is the consumer price index.

> **wage index**   A component used by the Health Care Financing Administration (HCFA) in adjusting payments (prices) under the Medicare prospective payment system (PPS). The wage index is derived by HCFA starting with data supplied by hospitals in response to a questionnaire; it takes into account normal work hours, as well as part-time and overtime work hours.

> **rural area wage index**   A wage index computed by Medicare for hospitals it classifies as rural hospitals.

indigent   Lacking the necessities of life; not having sufficient resources. "Indigent" will have different definitions for different purposes; for example, to qualify for a public assistance program.

medically indigent   The condition, as defined by the federal, state, or local government, of lacking the financial ability to pay for one's medical care. Any individual whose income and other resources falls below the defined level is declared to be medically "medically indigent"indigent and may qualify for public assistance.

indigent medical care (IMC)   Care for patients whose income falls below a level usually set by statute or regulation as defining indigency. Such care is provided without charge or for reduced charges, but the institution must find the resources by "overcharges" to other patients (or their payers), supplementary appropriations, public subscription, or elsewhere.

Indigo Institute   A 501(c)(3) organization which conducts and disseminates research on the organization, function, and financing of health care. The Institute explores innovative ways of changing the present health care system and thus the behavior of those who provide and those who receive care, so that communities may deliver health care with quality, in an efficient manner, for all. See also *Blue Indigo*.

individual health care account (IHCA)   A proposed method of financing health care costs by giving tax advantages to individuals who establish and maintain personal "individual health care accounts (ICHAs)" similar in concept to individual retirement accounts (IRAs). Money placed in such accounts would be excluded from the individual's taxable income and would be invested, with principal and income to be used only for specified health care. ICHAs could be a replacement for financing by Medicare for the elderly, a supplement to Medicare, or both. Synonym(s): health IRA, medical savings account (MSA) .

industry screening   See *blacklisting*.

infectious waste   See *hazardous waste*.

informatics   An emerging term (seeking a standard definition) which is used to cover information along with its management, particularly by computer. Usually the field involved is used along with "informatics," e.g., "medical informatics."

   medical informatics   A new discipline which covers medical (and related) information, both in traditional and electronic form, along with its management, particularly by computer methods. Included are the storage, retrieval, and use of the information (including, according to some authors, statistics).

information   A term generally used to mean data which have somehow been "digested" (manipulated, summarized, organized, or interpreted) so that inferences may more readily be drawn and decisions made than from "raw" data. See *data*.

information system   A poorly defined term used to refer to anything from a pencil and paper to a full-blown computer system. Usually the term "information system" is modified by words specifying its purpose, such as "management information system (MIS)."

   case mix management information system (case mix MIS)   An information system which combines and correlates, on an individual patient basis, medical data abstracted from the hospital medical record of the patient (discharge abstract) and from the patient's bill. Data analyses and displays relate charges, by Diagnosis

Related Groups (DRGs), to receipts or allowances for those DRGs for the hospital and for individual physicians. A case mix MIS may be provided in-house, off-site, or through shared services. See also *case mix.*

community health integrated management information system (CHIMIS) A set of computer systems and communication devices extending throughout the community in order to facilitate the exchange of clinical, financial, and management information among all parties involved: physicians, hospitals, schools, pharmacies, employers, and others involved in health and health care. The system provides continuous communication linkage among all the components of the entire health care system, so that the information for the care of patients is available where it is needed and when it is needed. Cost of care is reduced as is the cost of information management. The savings in both instances reflecting the minimizing of delays and the elimination of duplication in record-keeping.

Such a system is in operation in Milwaukee, and others are in various stages of development and testing. A CHIMIS is an extension throughout the community of the concept of the hospital's integrated management information system (IMIS).

hospital information system (HIS) A term applied to any system in a hospital dealing with information, usually with a computer involved. The kinds of data carried in the system will vary from hospital to hospital; there is no agreement yet on criteria which a system must meet to carry this title. An HIS is one kind of management information system (MIS).

integrated management information system (IMIS) A management information system which includes in its scope (integrates into a single system) management information from all elements of an enterprise.

management information system (MIS) An essentially undefined term, applied to any system set up to provide information to or for management. There is no agreement on the kinds of information to be carried or the technology used. The term "MIS" often implies that a computer is involved—sometimes the hospital's computer system, sometimes shared services with outside computers, and sometimes a hospital discharge abstract system. The information may include data on, for example, patients, finance, personnel, production, or the health care industry.

information technology (IT) The use of computers and computer applications to handle large masses of data. Information technology became a popular descriptive label during the 1990's, particularly among universities who wanted a broader label than "computer science" as a name for newly created departments that dealt with the explosion of computer usage.

infoweaver One who weaves a cohesive web of information from disparate bits of data and other information. This term was coined to extend the usual terms of "writer" and "editor". An infoweaver is a knowledgeworker whose skills include the ability to add hypertext links to written text, and to make the presentation of information interactive with its intended consumers. Infoweavers use not only text to present information, but also still and moving pictures, as well as sound, where appropriate. Synonym: multimedia author/editor.

injury (bodily)   The damage caused by an external force, as contrasted with an "illness," which simply indicates that the body is not in a healthy condition.

injury (legal)   The damage caused by a legal wrong. For example, defamation causes "injury" to a person's reputation; a breach of contract may cause financial injury.

in-network   An adjective applied to a provider or a service when the provider is a part of the health care network (or system) or the service is available within the network, and thus the cost has been the subject of prior agreement. The antonym is, of course, "out-of-network."

inpatient   A patient who receives care while being lodged in an institution.

Institute for Diversity in Health Management (IDHM)   An institute sponsored by the American Hospital Association (AHA), the America College of Healthcare Executives (ACHE), and the National Association of Health Services Executives (NAHSE) created in 1994 to inform minority students about opportunities in health care management and to assist ethnic minority professionals already in the field.

institution for mental diseases (IMD)   As defined by the Department of Health and Human Services (DHHS) for Medicaid, "an institution that is primarily engaged in providing diagnosis, treatment or care of persons with mental diseases." A hospital, skilled nursing facility (SNF), or intermediate care facility (ICF), for example, can also be an IMD for Medicaid purposes; the "overall character" of the institution governs.

institutional review board (IRB)   A committee in an investigator's institution set up to provide peer review for research programs supported by grants and contracts financed by the Department of Health and Human Services (DHHS). Similar review is also required by the Food and Drug Administration (FDA) for investigational new drugs. The committee may not have as members any persons who have professional responsibility in the conduct of the research. The research proposal is reviewed in terms of institutional commitments and regulations, applicable law, standards of professional conduct and practice, and community attitudes. The committee also is to ensure that informed consent of subjects is obtained by adequate and appropriate methods, whether or not the research involves risk to the subjects.

instructional advance directive (IAD)   See *instructional advance directive (IAD)* under *advance directive.*

insurance   A method of providing for money to pay for specific types of losses which may occur. Insurance is a contract (the insurance policy) between one party (the insured) and another (the insurer). The policy states what types of losses (see *risk*) are covered, what amounts will be paid for each loss and for all losses, and under what conditions.

Two types of insurance commonly spoken of in health care are: (1) insurance covering the patient for health care services (health insurance, also called a "third party payer"); and (2) insurance covering the health care provider for risks associated with the delivery of health care (liability to a patient for malpractice, for example).

captive insurance company   An insurance company formed to underwrite (insure) the risks of its owner(s). Increasingly, hospitals and other health care providers are forming or buying their own insurance companies, either alone or with other providers.

catastrophic insurance   Insurance intended to protect against the cost of a catastrophic illness, with "catastrophic" defined as exceeding a predetermined cost. Catastrophic insurance comes into play above that cost, in supplement of other insurance, and pays all or a percentage of the cost above the specified amount. Synonym(s): major medical insurance.

commercial insurance   In health care, usually any insurance for hospital or medical care other than that written by Blue Cross and Blue Shield (BC/BS) (which, so long as they remain nonprofit organizations, are "non-commercial").

general liability insurance   Insurance which covers the risk of loss for most accidents and injuries to third parties (the insured and its employees are not covered) which arise from the actions or negligence of the insured, and for which the insured may have legal liability, except those injuries directly related to the provision of professional health care services (the latter risks are covered by professional liability insurance).   General liability insurance will pay for slips and falls of visitors on hospital premises, for example.

health insurance   Insurance which covers the patient for health care, including physician and hospital services.

major medical insurance   See *catastrophic insurance*, above.

MediGap insurance   See *Medicare supplement insurance.*

out-of-area insurance   Insurance carried by a health care plan (such as an HMO) to pay for care for beneficiaries when they are away from home, away from the service area of the plan ("out-of-area").

professional liability insurance   Insurance which covers the risk of loss from patient injury or illness which results from professional negligence (see *negligence*) or other professional liability (see *liability (legal)*). Professional liability insurance pays malpractice claims. Often, a hospital's professional liability policy will not cover the actions of physicians on the medical staff, in which case those physicians need to obtain their own individual policies.

property insurance   Insurance which pays for damage to the insured's own property, for example, loss by fire.

self-insurance   Assumption of risk of loss without an insurance policy. For example, a hospital deciding to "self-insure" would set aside its own funds to protect itself against financial loss, instead of purchasing an insurance policy from an insurance company. In many cases, however, even a so-called "self-insured" hospital will purchase a policy (see *excess coverage*; under *insurance coverage*) to protect against very large losses. For example, a hospital might self-insure for losses up to three million dollars, then have a policy to cover the next ten million dollars of loss.

stop-loss insurance   Insurance carried by a health care plan, purchased from an insurance carrier, to reimburse the health care plan for costs of care for individual patients over a ceiling (for example, $10,000).

insurance benefits   See *benefits*.

insurance claim form   The form on which a physician or other provider submits the claim for care given. Each insurance company may design and require its own form, as can the federal and state governments. This lack of standardization has at least two negative consequences: everyone has to work much harder to complete and understand the form, and, automating this tedious task becomes much more difficult, if not impossible.

insurance coverage   Generally refers to the amount of protection available and the kind of loss which would be paid for under an insurance contract.

claims-made coverage   Insurance that will pay for claims which are made during the period of time that the policy is in effect, for events which occur *after* the insurance policy's retroactive date. For example, if a hospital has a claims-made insurance policy in effect for calendar year 1990, with a retroactive date of January 1, 1987, and a patient suffers an injury during a 1988 surgical procedure but does not notify (or sue) the hospital until 1990, the claim will be covered under the 1990 policy. If the surgery was in 1986, it will not be covered. See also *occurrence-based coverage*.

excess coverage   Extra high limits of insurance coverage, which will pay amounts over and above the original limits of a specified policy.

first-dollar coverage   Insurance which has no copayment or deductible provision; the insured does not have to pay the first dollar—the insurer pays it.

occurrence-based coverage   Insurance which will pay for claims only when the event which gives rise to the claim happens during the period of time that the policy is in effect, regardless of when the claim is made. For example, if a hospital has an occurrence-based insurance policy in effect only for calendar year 1990, and a patient suffers an injury during a 1988 surgical procedure, the claim will not be covered under the 1990 policy because the injury did not occur in 1990. See also *claims-made coverage*.

tail coverage   Insurance purchased to protect the insured after the end of a claims-made policy, to cover events which occurred during the period of the claims-made policy, but for which no claim was made during that period. This protects the insured in case a claim is made at a future date, after the original policy has lapsed. Sometimes this is referred to simply as a "tail."

umbrella coverage   A broad high limit liability policy, usually requiring underlying insurance. For example, a hospital may be insured for one million dollars for general liability and three million dollars for professional liability, with an umbrella of ten million dollars. The umbrella will pick up any excess liability over either policy, up to the ten million dollar additional limit.

wraparound coverage   Provides members of basic health care plans with coverage for certain services provided by non-plan providers. Beneficiaries of this type of supplemental insurance coverage are frequently members of HMO's or Medicare.

integrated delivery network (IDN)   See *integrated health delivery network (IHDN)*.

integrated delivery system (IDS)   See *integrated health delivery network (IHDN)*.

integrated health delivery network (IHDN)   A group of hospitals, physicians, other providers, insurers, and/or community agencies that work together to coordinate and deliver a broad spectrum of services to their community. This definition is from the *1995-96 AHA Guide*, which has for the first time a listing of "integrated health delivery networks." The *Guide* notes that it has identified networks of "varying organization type," and that the network listing is not mutually exclusive of the hospital, health care system, or alliance listings. IHDNs listed are representative of those in the lead or hub of network activity.

The amorphousness of the network definition is demonstrated by this caution from the *Guide*: "Networks are very fluid in their composition as goals evolve and partners change. Therefore, some of the networks included in this listing may have dissolved, reformed, or simply been renamed as this section was being produced for publication."

integrated health network   See *integrated health delivery network (IHDN)*.

integrated management information system (IMIS)   See *integrated management information system (MIS)* under *information system*.

integrated provider   See *integrated health delivery network (IHDN)*.

Integrated Services Digital Network (ISDN)   The telephone system of the future. ISDN is a technology which permits transmission of data on telephone lines at an extremely high speed, roughly 27 times faster than traditional technology. It uses digital signals instead of analog, and is therefore very popular among users who use telephone lines to connect computers to each other. Because of the digital signals, greatly improved audio quality is possible over phone lines. Availability of this service is dependent on your local phone company. Unfortunately by the mid 1990's many geographical areas still did not have ISDN, or it was prohibitively expensive. About the only drawback to ISDN is that it will require new telephones to take advantage of it.

integration   Integration is spoken of in health care today in terms of the linking together of components of the health care system:

horizontal integration   A linkage of hospitals (or other institutions and organizations) which are more or less alike, such as acute general hospitals, to form a multihospital system. The purpose of horizontal integration is to achieve economies of scale in operation, such as greater purchasing power and avoidance of duplication of facilities.

vertical integration   A linkage of hospitals (and other institutions and organizations) to form a system providing a range or continuum of care such as preventive, outpatient, acute hospital, long-term, home, and hospice care. The purpose of vertical integration is to keep the patient population within the one system for as many of its health care needs as possible.

interactive   Requiring or allowing a response from the user. In computer and telecommunications usage, interactive refers to a program that assumes the user or viewer will exercise some degree of choice to determine how the program will proceed. Almost all computer programs are interactive in that they present some kind of menu to the user, and then simply wait for the user's input. Almost all television programs now are not interactive, in that they are simply broadcast at a certain time, and the viewer either watches them or not. An interactive television program, for instance, might allow the user to click either of two buttons during the presentation of a movie, one called "Happy Ending" and the other "Sad Ending". You get to watch what you want to see, and the television company instantly knows not only who is watching their program, but what kind of ending they prefer. There are obviously many ramifications to interactive telecommunications that will need to be sorted out over time.

intergenerational dialog   Discussion in which several generations consider issues and problems from their respective points of view. When the young people in a community meet with senior citizens to discuss problems, the dialog is intergenerational.

intermediary   See *fiscal intermediary*.

International Classification of Clinical Services (ICCS)   A classification and coding system developed by the Commission on Professional and Hospital Activities (CPHA) for certain hospital-provided services in order to standardize patient care data and to facilitate computer handling of those data. Schemas are available for laboratory services, diagnostic imaging, and drugs. Similar schemas are under development for supplies, anesthesia, cardiology, respiratory therapy, physical medicine, nursing, and other categories.

International Classification of Diseases (ICD)   A publication of the World Health Organization (WHO), revised periodically, and now in its 9th Revision, dated 1975. The full title is *The International Classification of Diseases, Injuries, and Causes of Death*. This classification, which originated for use in classifying deaths, is used world-wide for that purpose. In addition, it has been used widely in the United States for hospital diagnosis classification since about 1955 through adaptations and modifications made in the United States of the 7th, 8th, and 9th Revisions. Modification was required for hospital use since, as discussed under *classification*, the purpose of the classification determines the pigeonholes; for example, "death pigeonholes" are quite different, in many instances, from those for illnesses and injuries. The modification in current use, the International Classification of Diseases, Ninth Revision, Clinical Modification (ICD-9-CM), published in 1978, has been in official use in the United States since 1979.

The 10th Revision, released in 1994, contains additional reasons why people seek help from, and how they are affected by, both the public health programs and the health care systems of the world. Its title will be the International Statistical Classification of Diseases and Related Health Problems.

International Classification of Diseases, Ninth Revision, Clinical Modification (ICD-9-CM)   The classification in current use for coding of diagnoses and operations for indexing medical records by diagnoses and operations, for compiling hospital statistics, and for submitting bills in the prospective payment system (PPS). *ICD-9-CM* is published by the Commission on Professional and Hospital Activities (CPHA) and by the federal government. *Annotated ICD-9-CM*, published by CPHA, is a version color-coded to alert users to reimbursement-related issues.

Internet (The Net)   A worldwide network of computer networks that can share information because a common set of language protocols ("TCP/IP") are used by all. Having origins similar to America's interstate highway system, the Internet was created in the interests of national defense by the US government. Begun by Vinton Cerf and Robert Kahn in the early 1970's to allow military computers to talk reliably to university research computers, the Internet has grown ever since. In the 1990's the Internet caught the public's fancy and the growth rate exploded. Up to this point there had been an understanding that the Internet was to be used only for *non-profit* enterprises such as research, but by the mid-1990's it had clearly become a free-for-all venture, with over 20 million users in over 175 countries. As this is being written in 1995, it must be said the Internet is clearly going through all the usual growing pains of any organization of this magnitude, and tomorrow's Internet will be different from today's.

Contrary to the belief of many, and certainly running against the hype of the media, the Internet is not an "official" organization with a centralized management plan, or even rules of conduct. While the concept of "netiquette" (be a good neighbor) is encouraged, the Internet is definitely more akin to the Wild West before US Marshals came on the scene. Following the tradition of the frontier, the Internet is now being populated by the farmers, ranchers, and miners for whom profit is an important consideration. It is to be expected that some form of governance will evolve if the Internet is to survive the coming years. In the meantime, there is gold to be found on the Internet, but mining is still hard work for most.

One of the difficulties encountered in finding any information on the Internet is the almost total lack of organization and standardization in how information is stored. There is no Dewey Decimal System directing you to a particular aisle or stack. One of the only rules is that each node on this worldwide inter-network must have a unique address, much like a phone number. A typical address in computer form may look like "198.87.128.43", but thanks to the *Domain Name System (DNS)* (which see), this address may resolve itself into a form more understandable by humans such as "tringa.com". This address is known as the computer's "Uniform Resource Locator (URL)". Most computers today have mass storage devices requiring that data be organized in subdirectories under the top (home) directory, and these various layers of subdirectories also become part of the URL. If you've ever used a computer with a hard disk, you realize now how many possible places there are to store (and lose track of) information. There is at least a partial solution that comes in the form of software designed to help you find things. Often called by names such as "web crawlers" or spiders, these programs literally spend their waking hours going from URL to URL, taking notes about what they find there. These notes are then digested and stored, and when coupled with a search engine, allow you, the user, to enter a search string and be presented with a list of "hits". This sounds good in theory, and in fact does work better than the impossible alternative of searching manually, but it's still a far cry from what we've come to expect in terms of the "library" metaphor, where information is organized in a coherent system to begin with.

A major factor in the Internet's explosive growth has been the rise of "multimedia". Information on the Internet traditionally was in text form, stored in files which would be transferred from one site to another, and read by the receiver. Now, the Internet is being used to store and transmit sights and sounds as well as text, making the information more appealing to a greater audience. Limited only by bandwidth, the Internet can carry live telephone-type conversations, including the transmission of live video of the persons carrying on the conversation. The potential here for health care is vast, ranging from broader access to health information to such things as patients being 'seen' by doctors remotely.

While the bulk of attention is focused on the "world wide web" (WWW, or just "the web") part of the Internet, the Net also supports "telnet" for terminal type connections to other computers; "ftp" (file transfer protocol) for the efficient transfer of files between computers, and other programs and utilities.

Included among the thousands of computer networks involved in The Net are the citizen-operated computer bulletin board systems (BBSs), the United States National Research and Education Network (NREN), COARA and TWICS in Japan, CIX in England, Usenet (worldwide), GlasNet in the former Soviet Union, Calva-Com in Europe, PeaceNet, EcoNet, and others.

interrater reliability   See *interrater reliability* under *reliability*.

Interstudy   A nonprofit health care research body, a "think tank," located in Minneapolis, Minnesota.

intrapreneur   A person *within* an organization who creates a new venture or "product" for the organization, as contrasted with an "entrepreneur," a person who organizes a new venture and assumes the risk.

intrarater reliability   See *intrarater reliability* under *reliability*.

inurement   Private gain from corporate activities. A nonprofit corporation (see *corporation*) cannot keep its tax exempt status if there is "inurement" to individuals or proprietary (for-profit) interests. One common area in which inurement issues are raised today is physician recruitment. Hospitals often provide incentives to attract physicians in needed specialties. If the hospital contracts to pay the physician a salary in excess of reasonable compensation for services, or provides an interest-free loan to the physician, these incentives may be considered by the Internal Revenue Service (IRS) to be inurement and thus jeopardize the hospital's tax exempt status. The hospital must show that it (and the community) receive measurable value for the incentives provided. Inurement issues are also sometimes raised by hospital joint ventures.

involuntary smoking   Inhaling air containing tobacco smoke produced by other persons who are smoking. It is also called passive smoking. Synonym(s): passive smoking.

J

Jackson Hole Group   An informal "think tank" founded by Paul Elwood, MD, President of Interstudy, in the early 1970s. Elwood convenes a small group of persons interested in the problems they perceive in the health care system at his home in Jackson Hole, Wyoming, and leads informal discussions on possible solutions to the problems. Their commitment is to "shaping sensible, market-based health care reform in the U.S." A total of nearly 90 individuals have participated in the discussions, now held about every three months, although any given meeting is limited to about twenty invited persons. The three constant members are Elwood, Alain Enthoven, Stanford University health economist, and Lynn Etheredge, Washington, DC, based consultant. The group gained national attention with the 1991 release of a "white paper" entitled "The 21st Century American Health System: The Jackson Hole Group Proposals for Health Care Reform Through Managed Competition."

JCAHO   See *Joint Commission on Accreditation of Healthcare Organizations.*

job lock   Remaining in employment for fear of losing one's health insurance coverage. This is caused by waiting periods for pre-existing conditions, high rates, and outright denials of coverage.

jocko   A common pronunciation of the acronym JCAHO. See *Joint Commission on Accreditation of Healthcare Organizations (JCAHO).*

Joint Commission on Accreditation of Healthcare Organizations (JCAHO)   An independent, nonprofit, voluntary organization sponsored by the American College of Physicians (ACP), the American College of Surgeons (ACS), the American Hospital Association (AHA), the American Medical Association (AMA), and other medical, dental, and health care organizations. JCAHO is the successor to the Hospital Standardization Program (HSP) of the ACS. It is based in Chicago, Illinois. Governance is by a Board of Commissioners designated by the sponsoring organizations.

JCAHO develops standards and provides accreditation surveys and certification to hospitals and to other health care organizations, such as psychiatric facilities, long-term care facilities, ambulatory care, and hospital care. It also offers education programs, consultation, and publications. It should be noted that the JCAHO Accreditation Manual for Hospitals (AMH), published annually, has a glossary defining terms as used by JCAHO. The JCAHO is often referred to simply as the Joint Commission. It was formerly (until 1987) called the Joint Commission on Accreditation of Hospitals (JCAH).

joint conference committee A hospital committee with members from the governing body, the medical staff, and the hospital management (administration). Its purpose is to facilitate understanding and communication, not to introduce a channel of management which competes with the line channels of the hospital administration and the medical staff.

joint planning See *joint planning* under *planning*.

joint venture A business arrangement between two or more parties to share profits, losses, and control. In health care, the term usually indicates a formalized cooperative effort between the hospital and its medical staff (or physicians from its medical staff), as opposed to a relationship in which the two, hospital and physicians, are in competition with one another. For example, a joint venture may be established in order to set up a diagnostic facility.

The legal form of the joint venture may be a partnership (general or limited), lease arrangement, corporation, or other form suited to the requirements of the venture. Sometimes the term "joint venture" is used synonymously with "partnership"; however, while a partnership may be a joint venture, not all joint ventures are partnerships. "Joint venture" may also have a specific legal meaning under state law.

Joint ventures may raise legal concerns for hospitals; see *antitrust*, *fraud and abuse*, *inurement*, and *safe harbor regulations*.

K

KDB See *knowledge database* under *database*.

Kaiser-Permanente Short for Kaiser-Permanente Medical Care Program, America's largest private health care system, and considered to be a pioneer in comprehensive prepayment systems. It includes the following three components:

(1) Kaiser Foundation Health Plan, the health maintenance organization (HMO) under which the members are organized. In July 1993, Kaiser HMOs based in San Francisco and Los Angeles, each with over 2 million members, were top ranked by *Money* magazine. The San Francisco HMO was started in 1945.

(2) Kaiser Foundation Hospitals, a nonprofit corporation that provides the hospital services to the HMO members. According to the American Hospital Association's *Guide to the Health Care Field*, this component had 29 hospitals (6,151 beds) in 1994, in California, Hawaii, and Oregon.

(3) The Permanente Medical Groups, the physician partnerships and professional corporations which provide the actual medical services to the HMO.

knowledge asymmetry The situation which exists when two individuals are attempting to come to a decision and the amount of information each has on the subject is very different. For example, until recent developments, physicians have had far more information on diseases and their treatment than patients, and attempts to empower patients to participate in decision-making on their own care have been largely futile. See *Health Commons Institute (HCI), decision support software (DSS), informed consent, shared decision making,* and *problem knowledge couplers.*

knowledge-based   Supported by actual, relevant information. Knowledge used here means data. In health care, "knowledge" specifically means data about a particular population rather than generalizations about typical populations. The specific population may be that of a geographic community or that for which a given health care provider (HMO, MCO, physician) is responsible. The data are of two kinds: demographic data and performance data.

The demographic data begins with the usual items: the size of the population and its age and sex distribution, and vital statistics including mortality and morbidity. To these are added such data as can be obtained about the population's special health and environmental characteristics, ethnic makeup, and sources of payment for health care.

When the population under consideration is that served by a health care provider, data on the performance of that provider can be added to the "knowledge base." This requires a management information system which carries the necessary detail about diagnoses, procedures, and patient care management, and thus permits compilations of statistical patterns on such items as immunizations given, use of hospital days, surgical and other treatments, use of prescription drugs, and so on. The data can be used to develop report cards for individual physicians and other caregivers and institutions. Comparisons of these patterns against recognized standards, the performance of peers, and against benchmark data are useful in managing and improving practices.

Such a system can sometimes provide contemporaneous patient safeguards, in addition to retrospective analysis and future planning. In the more sophisticated systems, which employ online analytical processing (OLAP), rules are developed (rudimentary artificial intelligence) by which one component of the computer processing is a continuous monitoring of performance. Warning alarms are sounded in "real time" for individual patients when predetermined signal events (usually dangerous) are detected. For example, it is common for a warning to sound when an order is issued for a drug incompatible with another already being given, or for a drug for which dietary restrictions should be invoked.

L

LAN   See *local area network.*

legacy system   A computer term referring to an inherited set of independent computer systems within an organization (enterprise). The term comes into use as enterprises seek to consolidate the systems of the past into a single information source, either by somehow linking them together so that they can communicate with each other (and with the inquirer) or, more likely, by replacing them with an integrated management information system (IMIS) (see *information system*). Hospitals commonly have installed at different times independent computer systems for laboratory, X-ray, business office, and admitting, for example. Unless this legacy system is replaced by an IMIS, (1) it is impossible to obtain a comprehensive view of the hospital's activities, (2) since much of the same information is found in each system, such as patient demographic data, there is a much higher likelihood of error than if there were a single entry for each piece of information, and (3) there is duplication of cost. Legacy system is also frequently used to describe *any* previously existing computer system that is considered to be now obsolete and ready for replacement, or incorporation into a new system.

length of stay (LOS) The number of days between a patient's admission and discharge. The day of admission is counted as a day, while the day of discharge is not. This abbreviation is often misused when the intent is to refer to average length of stay (ALOS).

average length of stay (ALOS) A standard hospital statistic. For a given group of patients, their total lengths of stay (see *length of stay (LOS)*) are added together, and that total is divided by the total number of patients in the group. For a "hospital ALOS," the formula adds together the LOSs of all patients discharged from the hospital (for their entire stays) in a given time period, and divides that sum by the number of patients discharged in that same time period. ALOS is often incorrectly referred to as "LOS"; however, LOS means "length of stay" and pertains to an individual patient.

The ALOS may be calculated not only for the entire hospital, but also for specific age groups or Diagnosis Related Groups (DRGs), for example. It may also be calculated in a more refined ("normalized") manner by making an adjustment for the case mix of the hospital. An ALOS which adjusts for the age distribution of the patients, for example, makes for fairer comparisons between hospitals than one without such an adjustment; adjusting for additional factors, such as the distribution of patients among DRGs, further improves the statistic for interhospital comparison purposes.

level of care The amount (intensity) and kind of professional nursing care required for a patient in order to achieve the desired medical and nursing care objectives for the patient, that is, to carry out the orders of the attending physician and to meet the patient's nursing care needs. The term "level of care" is primarily used outside the acute hospital, where three levels of care are recognized: skilled nursing care (the highest level), intermediate care, and rest home care (custodial care, the lowest level).

Levels of care (and facilities to provide them) have specific definitions in Medicare, Medicaid, and other payment programs, and also under statutes and regulations of the various states. The determination of the level of care to be provided to a given patient is a serious matter; on the one hand, the patient should be placed at the lowest level of care commensurate with his needs as a matter both of appropriate care and of economy, while, on the other hand, payment is greater for each succeedingly higher level of care.

leverage Financing by borrowing.

capital leverage See *financial leverage*.

financial leverage   The ratio of total debt to total assets (in a stock corporation, the ratio of long-term debt to shareholders' equity). Financial leverage is also called "capital leverage." An institution uses financial leverage (it "trades on its equity") when it believes it has "positive leverage," that is, that it can use the money obtained by debt financing (see *financing*) to earn more money than it costs to borrow the money (interest and taxes). Should the cost of borrowing exceed the added revenue, the situation is one of "negative leverage."

negative leverage   See *financial leverage*.

operating leverage   The ratio of fixed costs to variable costs (see *cost*). When it takes very little added labor or materials to provide added units of service or products, the operating leverage is high (and the marginal cost of added units is low); a greater volume brings accelerated profits, once the break-even point is reached. The higher the proportion of the costs that are variable (that is, the lower the operating leverage) the greater an increase in units of service or products will be required to increase profits.

positive leverage   See *financial leverage*.

leveraged   Financed largely by borrowed funds. See *leverage*.

liability (legal)   Responsibility to do something, pay something, or refrain from doing something. Liability is used to refer to a legal obligation, often one which must be enforced by a lawsuit.

corporate liability   Legal responsibility of a corporation, rather than of an individual. In the health care context, the term is often used to denote a specific type of responsibility: that of the hospital as an institution (corporation) to exercise reasonable care in selecting, retaining, and granting privileges to members of its medical staff. A hospital may be liable to a patient injured by a physician (or other health professional) if the hospital knew or should have known that the physician was not competent to perform the procedure involved (or to otherwise treat the patient), and did not reasonably act to protect the patient (for example, by restricting that physician's privileges or by requiring supervision). "Knew" means that the hospital may not "look the other way" if it learns of problems with a physician which could endanger patients; "should have known" means that the hospital must diligently investigate a physician's credentials prior to granting staff privileges, *and* that the hospital must systematically monitor the care provided by that physician, once on the staff.

enterprise liability   A system under which individual health care providers are relieved of liability for medical malpractice, and health care organizations such as hospitals and health maintenance organizations bear liability for malpractice committed by their affiliated care providers, whether or not those providers are employees of the organization. The system is proposed by Kenneth S. Abraham, JD, Class of 1962 Professor of Law, University of Virginia School of Law. Sometimes called "organizational liability."

joint and several liability   The responsibility of more than one defendant to share in legal liability to a plaintiff. If the defendants (for example, the hospital and a physician) are jointly and severally liable, each is responsible to pay the entire judgment to the plaintiff (although the plaintiff cannot collect more than the amount of the judgment).

product liability   An area of law which imposes legal responsibility on manufacturers (and in some cases distributors and retailers) of goods which leave the factory in an unreasonably dangerous condition, and which in fact cause harm to someone because of that condition. Product liability does not require proof that the manufacturer was negligent (careless) in designing or producing the item.

professional liability   A legal obligation which is the result of performing (or failing to perform) something which one does (or should have done) as a professional. A physician who drives carelessly and injures another will be simply "liable" for that person's injuries; the fact that she is a physician is not relevant to the fact that she injured the other person. If that same physician carelessly misses a diagnosis and again injures another, the legal responsibility is called "professional liability," since her actions as a physician caused the injury. Sometimes the phrase "professional liability" is used interchangeably with "professional negligence," but that usage is inaccurate because a professional can become liable for reasons other than negligence (for example, by improperly disclosing a patient's confidences, operating without informed consent, or abandoning a patient).

strict liability   Legal responsibility for injury which is imposed regardless of any fault, or lack of fault. A plaintiff suing under strict liability does not need to show that the defendant was negligent, reckless, or malicious. The plaintiff does, however, still need to prove the existence of a defect (such as in a product) or an action (such as selling liquor to an intoxicated person) and that the defect or action caused the plaintiff's injuries.

liability (financial)   In finance, an obligation to pay. Liabilities are shown on an institution's balance sheet under such headings as "accounts payable" (money owed to vendors and others), "accrued salaries" (when a statement is drawn before checks have been issued for a given pay period), and the like.

current liability   A liability due within one year.

licensed   Having a legal right, granted by a government agency, in compliance with a statute governing a profession (such as medicine or nursing), occupation, or the operation of an activity (such as a hospital).

licensed beds   See *licensed beds* under *bed capacity*.

licensed health care professional   See *licensed health care professional* under *professional*.

life care   A long-term care arrangement ("alternative") in which all care required for the lifetime of the participant is provided. A retirement home which agrees to provide not only facilities for independent living, but also nursing care and hospitalization to residents as needed, is a "life care community."

life expectancy   A statistically-derived estimate as to how much longer a given individual may be expected to live. Reference tables for life expectancy have been produced by insurance companies and public health statisticians for many years. The earliest such tables took into account age- and sex-specific death rates compiled for the general population, usually by governmental offices of vital statistics. The tables are periodically updated as these offices publish new data, and the more recent tables have been refined as data has become available permitting adjustments for other factors, such as smoking habits, occupation, and family history.

life support   Maintenance of vital body functions, e.g. breathing and heartbeat, to sustain life.

life support system   Equipment and services, including administration of nutrition and fluids, which support one or more of the life-sustaining functions of circulation (heart), respiration (breathing), nutrition, and kidney function. When a patient is completely dependent on artificial (mechanical) means for maintenance of one or more of these functions, stopping or removing the equipment will cause death, and the stopping or removal is referred to as "termination of life support systems."

lifetime reserve   A Medicare term referring to the pool of 60 days of hospital care upon which a patient may draw after she has used up the maximum Medicare benefit for a single spell of illness.

liquidity   The ability to turn assets into cash.

living-in unit   A hospital room where a mother can assume care of her newborn infant under the supervision of the hospital's nursing personnel. This term may also apply to relatives or others assisting in the care of a chronically ill or other type of patient.

living will   See *living will* under *advance directive*.

lobbying   Attempts to influence the passage or defeat of legislation. There are limits on such activities, and certain other political activities, by tax-exempt organizations, such as 501(c)(3) corporations. Hospitals are often tax-exempt 501(c)(3) organizations, and thus are limited in their lobbying (and campaigning) efforts.

local area network (LAN)   The hardware and software allowing two or more computers to be connected together over a small geographic area (typically an office, or one building). It is distinguished from a "wide area network" (WAN) which connects computers, other networks, or both over large geographical distances.

  LANs are becoming increasingly important in allowing microcomputers (personal computers, PCs) to be connected to each other. LANs allow PC users to share data and resources which once required the use of mini or mainframe computers. A major stumbling block to even greater acceptance of LAN technology is the lack of standards in network protocols. By the mid 1990's however, the remaining network vendors had largely implemented methods by which most computers could communicate with each other in spite of differing protocols.

local health department   A unit of local government which is the action arm of national and state public health agencies. It typically carries out some clinical services, environmental services, and support services. Clinical services may include, for example, dental health, occupational health, nursing, maternal and child health, family planning, communicable disease, and Women, Infants and Children's Programs (WIC). Environmental services may include general environment, vector control, animal control, and pollution control. Support services may include, in addition to administration, vital statistics, laboratory, and health education.

locality rule A legal doctrine which states that the standard of care (legal) in a malpractice lawsuit will be measured by the degree of care exercised by similar professionals within the same geographic area (locality), rather than within the world, nation, state, or profession at large. Some states use this rule; others do not.

long-term care (LTC) Care for patients, regardless of age, who have chronic diseases or disabilities, and who require preventive, diagnostic, therapeutic, and supportive services over long periods of time. LTC may call on a variety of health care professionals (such as physicians, nurses, physical therapists, and social workers) as well as non-professionals (family, others) and may be delivered in a health care or other institution or in the home.

Long-term care customarily refers to those for whom the care is thought to be necessary for the rest of their lives, i.e., for whom the disability is thought not to be reversible. When the prediction is that the person can be returned to a more independent mode of living, the person is placed under skilled nursing or intermediate care (under "extended care" rather than "long-term care"); see *nursing care*. Rehabilitation efforts are, however, made for persons in long-term care, and some of them do recover sufficiently to become less dependent.

long-term care facility (LTCF) A facility which provides lodging and health care services to patients with chronic health care needs.

LOS See *length of stay*.

loss (financial) Excess of expense over income. Actually means a decrease in assets. The defining phrase "negative fund balance" is often used in nonprofit corporations (see *corporation*) as a substitute for the word "loss."

loss (insurance) An amount an insurance company is obligated to pay under an insurance contract, usually due to physical damage or injury to the property or person of the insured or a third party.

loss ratio Total incurred claims for a given insurance plan divided by the total premiums.

M

macro measures In health care, refers to steps taken to improve the health care system at the community level (for example, local, state, or national) with respect to such problems as insurance, financing, tort reform, access, and the like, rather than care to individual patients. See also *micro measures*.

macroeconomics The economic theory which pertains to forces which determine the decisions and actions of populations, rather than of individuals. The latter theory is called microeconomics.

MADPA See *Medicaid Antidiscriminatory Drug Pricing and Patient Benefit Restoration Act*.

magnetic sitter An electronic system similar to that used in clothing stores to detect removal of a magnetically tagged garment past a sensor at the exit. Similar magnetic "sitters" are used to keep track of patients who, because of confusion, may wander away or enter a dangerous area. Such patients, who would otherwise have to be restrained, may be granted freedom of movement, with assurance that sensors placed near exits, windows, and other areas denied to patients will inform the nursing staff.

mainframe computer See *mainframe computer* under *computer*.

mainstreaming A policy of providing services to special classes of individuals within the organizational structure which serves the general population. For example, handicapped children, often educated in special classrooms, are "mainstreamed" when they are educated in the regular classroom. The term is now being applied in health care in some instances.

Major Diagnostic Category (MDC) A term used in the prospective payment system (PPS). All patients are ultimately classified into one of the 468 Diagnosis Related Groups (DRGs) (categories). On the way to that classification, each patient first falls into one of 23 MDCs on the basis of his principal diagnosis (see *diagnosis*); the patient is then further classified according to age, complications, whether an operating room procedure was performed, and so forth.

major medical insurance See *catastrophic insurance* under *insurance*.

malpractice A failure of care or skill by a professional, which causes loss or injury and results in legal liability. This narrow definition means the same as "professional negligence". Some use the term "malpractice" more broadly to describe all acts by a health care professional in the course of providing health care—including breach of contract—which may result in legal liability.

malpractice reform See *tort reform*.

managed care Any arrangement for health care in which someone is interposed between the patient and physician and has authority to place restraints on how and from whom the patient may obtain medical and health services, and what services are to be provided in a given situation. Under the terms of a prepaid health plan, for example, the payer may require: that except in an emergency, a designated person (usually a physician; see *gatekeeper*) be the patient's first contact with the health care services; that all care be authorized and coordinated by the gatekeeper rather than permitting the patient to go directly to specialists; that only certain physicians and facilities be used (if the prepayment plan is to pay for the services); that preadmission certification (PAC) precede hospitalization; that second opinions be obtained for elective surgery; and that certain care be delivered in the outpatient setting.

Managed care was originally designed to control costs, encourage efficient use of resources, and ensure that care given is appropriate. However, there is increasing interest in trying to see that each patient *gets* the care indicated and is spared unnecessary or ill-advised care.

managed care organization (MCO) A term applied to a variety of organizations which contract to provide management services for the reduction and control of health care costs to corporations, insurers, and third party administrators. MCOs employ such methods as making decisions as to what care is to be given individual patients and where it will be provided, negotiating contracts with providers as to quantities of and prices for services (often discounts), and auditing and approving the bills for the services the patients receive. Sometimes the MCO offers a stipulated care package for a prearranged capitation fee. Typically such organizations do not themselves provide care and do not operate hospitals or other health care facilities. They would, however, have legal obligations similar to those of *managed care plans*; see below.

managed care plan (MCP) An organization providing managed care. A managed care plan has a defined group of providers and an identified group of enrollees to be served. Forward-looking plans develop explicit standards of care to be required of its providers, and are concerned not only with treatment and amelioration of disease, but also with prevention. The plan may or may not operate its own hospitals or other health care facilities. The financing is typically prearranged by capitation.

There are different purposes for managed care plans. One is for-profit, to make money for shareholders of a corporation. Another is a non-profit plan set up by hospitals, physicians, insurers, or others, to control rising health care costs—to save money. Yet another may have as its primary purpose the preservation and improvement of the health of its members. A community may use managed care, for example, as a strategy to: (1) benefit the individuals served by the plan, (2) benefit the health of the entire community, and (3) provide services in the most efficient, effective, and economic manner in view of the finite resources available.

Perhaps the biggest concern about managed care is that people will not get the medical care they need. In fact, some plans are more concerned about patient care than others. However, it is becoming clear that a managed care plan—whether owned by an insurance company, hospital, or whatever—is in a fiduciary relationship with respect to the enrollees, and may not act in a manner which jeopardizes their welfare. For example, the North Carolina Court of Appeals recently held a hospital liable because it had a policy to discharge patients when their insurance ran out; that this interfered with the medical judgement of the physician; and that this resulted in the premature discharge of a psychiatric patient who later committed suicide. [Even though a managed care plan was not involved, the principles would be the same.]

managed competition (MC) A strategy for purchasing health care in a manner which, it is proposed, would obtain maximum value for the price for the purchasers of the health care and the recipients. The concept was developed primarily by Alain Enthoven (Stanford University), and has been promulgated by the Jackson Hole Group.

The strategy depends on the existence of "sponsors" and acceptable providers, under government regulation. Sponsors for certain groups already exist in the form of large employers, state governments, and similar institutions. For smaller and less well-organized groups, an organization called a "health alliance" (HA) is envisioned as the sponsor. The HA would be a nonprofit corporation established by appropriate employer and community groups. The sponsor would act as an intermediary between the population to be insured and the competing provider groups (accountable health plans (AHPs)) which take care of both financing and delivery of care. (For competition to occur, of course, there would need to be more than one supplier.)

The "competition" would be price competition among annual premiums for a defined, standardized benefit package rather than for individual services. The competition is to be "informed" in that the sponsor has data and expertise to guide it, along with an informed, critical population of subscribers being served. Presumably the AHP which convinces both the sponsor and the consumers that it can provide the highest quality of care, at the lowest cost, and with the most satisfied patients (beneficiaries), will flourish because of increased business.

The sponsor would (1) select participating AHPs; (2) make sure that the eligible providers (AHPs) cannot evade price competition; (3) take care of the enrollment process; (4) insist on equity, which includes such considerations as availability of the plan to every applicant (even though subsidy may be required), continuous coverage, community rating, and no exclusion for preexisting conditions; (5) make sure that the premium is adjusted on the basis of the risks presented by the covered population so that surcharges or subsidies, as may be required, are applied and result in equal premiums among the AHPs; and (6) make sure that the demand is price-elastic (that is, the more subscribers, the lower the cost).

Managed competition proponents make the following contentions: (1) MC is expected to work because it depends on the application of proven microeconomic principles; (2) pluralism is insured because of the existence of a choice of providers; (3) individuals are made responsible for their own health; and (4) all citizens are covered (although financing is not a component of the MC process). Proponents insist that managed competition is *not*: free market, a voucher system, deregulation, more of the present system, mandatory enrollment in HMOs or large clinics, lower quality care, a blind experiment, a "buzz-word" without definition, a panacea, or a process difficult to implement, requiring a long time to put in place.

management (Mx) (case)   The plan and course of action for the care of the patient, often shown in the shorthand "Mx", similar to "Dx" for diagnosis and "Rx," which is used for "treatment" as well as for "prescription."

management (organization)   In an organization, the task of getting things done systematically by, through, or with people with the necessary tools and facilities.

contract management   An arrangement under which an "employing" institution obtains ongoing management services from a "managing" organization under a contract. The employing institution retains full ownership of and final responsibility for the institution. The services to be rendered by the contracting organization are spelled out in the management contract.   If the contractual services are for department management, the contracting organization reports to the employing institution exactly as though its manager were the employing institution's own employee, that is, at the same point in the hierarchy. If the contractual services are for the management of the entire institution, the contracting organization furnishes a chief executive officer (CEO) who reports to the governing body of the employing institution as though he were employed by the governing body as its CEO. Contract management is one variety of relationship found in some multihospital systems.

product line management (PLM)   A type of management in which the organization is considered to be a cluster or assemblage of strategic business units (SBUs). Each SBU has a separate product with a distinct market. In a hospital, a specific operation or class of operations (for example, eye surgery) could be considered an SBU, as could an alcoholism rehabilitation service. Each SBU has its specific resource requirements, information system needs, and management demands. Hospitals try to determine which product lines are "saleable" in their service areas and for which they have appropriate resources, and which they feel put them in advantageous competitive positions, and concentrate on those product lines.

service management   A philosophy of management which emphasizes "service" to mean satisfaction of the demands and wishes of the customer and attention to his perceptions, rather than paying primary attention to the "products" provided or satisfying the provider (the hospital or physician, for example).

management information system (MIS)   See *management information system (MIS)* under *information system*.

manager   Any individual who is responsible for directing the activities of an organization or one of its components. In the hospital field, however, the title of "manager" is rarely given to high ranking persons, particularly in the professions; the chief executive officer (CEO) and the chief of nursing are not called "managers." The title is more likely to be used in such areas of the hospital as housekeeping, maintenance, and the like.

mandate   To require, or a requirement. In health care, the term is being used to refer to federal- or state-imposed requirements on insurance companies, employers, and so forth, to pay for health care or to provide specific benefits:

employer mandate   A requirement that employers must provide coverage for their employees or be penalized. Also called "play or else."

play or pay   A slang phrase describing a proposed employer mandate which would require the employer to either participate in the health care plan offered or pay for an acceptable alternative, such as a tax which would go to a public plan to provide for the employed uninsured and the unemployed. Synonym(s): "pay or play."

state mandate   State laws which mandate private health care insurers to cover a wide variety of services, including well baby care and so forth, sometimes resulting in premiums out of reach of small employers. See also *bare-bones health plan*.

mandatory assignment   A requirement for physicians to accept Medicare reimbursement as payment in full for their services; they would not be allowed to bill the patient for any difference between their fees and the amount that Medicare will pay.

marginal worker   See *contingent worker*.

market   The characteristics of the buyers of health services; also can mean the geographical area to which services are to be provided.

market-based approach   See *consumer choice*.

market-driven system   See *market-driven system* under *economic system*.

market forces   The economic forces of supply and demand.

marketing   Activity to publicize a hospital or service, and to increase its use. See also *demarketing*.

Marshfield Clinic case   A federal antitrust case in which the appellate opinion suggests that providers can freely deal with (or even refuse to deal with) insurance companies even where the providers have a "natural monopoly" (the market is just too small to support additional providers). At trial it was argued that a provider (Marshfield Clinic and its wholly-owned HMO) had violated federal antitrust laws by signing up virtually all of the physicians within its market area into its managed care program with exclusive contracts, thereby preventing an insurance company (Blue Cross & Blue Shield of Wisconsin and its HMO) from competing on a "level playing field." The jury in the original federal district court case agreed with Blue Cross and awarded them $48 million, after trial reduced to around $20 million. Virtually every issue at trial, however, was reversed in September 1995 by the Court of Appeals for the Seventh Circuit. Central to the appellate courts opinion was the conclusion that HMOs were not a separate or unique health care market in the area, but simply another way of pricing medical care, much like PPOs or other forms of managed care. *Blue Cross & Blue Shield of Wisconsin v. The Marshfield Clinic, No. 94-C-137-S (W.D. Wisc., October 28, 1994).*

materiel   The tools, equipment, and supplies necessary to do any given work, as contrasted with the personnel needed to do the work.

maternal and child health program (MCH program)   A program providing preventive and treatment services for pregnant women, mothers, and children. The services may include health education (often with particular attention to nutrition) and family planning. Funding may be from federal, state, or local sources. One source of funds has been the United States Maternal and Child Health Program under the Social Security Act.

maximum allowable actual charges (MAAC)   Limits for physician charge increases which were set by federal statute enacted in 1986. The statute applies only to physicians who are "non-participating" (that is, who have not agreed to accept the Medicare payment allowance as full payment). The limits apply to average charges, rather than charges for specific services; thus, compliance must be evaluated retrospectively, and enforcement is complicated.

McCarran-Ferguson Act   A 1945 act which declared that the insurance industry was not affected by federal laws regulating interstate commerce, unless the laws specifically applied to insurance. As a result, health care insurers have not been subject to federal antitrust laws. Some propose that the antitrust exemption for health care insurers should be repealed.

McKinney Homeless Assistance Act (MHAA)   A federal act passed in 1987 to fund health and social services for the homeless. Programs include physical and mental health care, substance abuse treatment, housing, shelter, outreach, education, job training, and social services. Current funding provides services for only about 15% of the nation's homeless.

mediation   A method of settling disputes by bringing the parties together to agree on a solution, rather than having a third party (such as an arbitrator, judge, or jury) make the decision for them. Mediation, usually done with the assistance of a mediator (someone trained in dispute resolution), may be private or may be connected to the court system. Some states have laws requiring or encouraging mediation as an alternative or supplement to costly, time-consuming lawsuits or trials.

Medicaid   The federal program which provides health care to indigent and medically indigent persons. While partially federally funded, the Medicaid program is administered by the states, in contrast with Medicare, which is federally funded and administered at the federal level. The Medicaid program was established in 1965 by amendment to the Social Security Act, under a provision entitled "Title XIX—Medical Assistance."

Medicaid Antidiscriminatory Drug Pricing and Patient Benefit Restoration Act (MADPA)   A federal law enacted in 1990 aimed at pharmaceutical cost containment. It requires drug companies to provide, through a rebate system, the "best prices" in the Medicaid outpatient pharmacy program. It also established a moratorium on reductions in pharmacy service reimbursement rates; guarantees Medicaid outpatients access to drug therapy consultations with their pharmacists; and requires review, in the outpatient program, of drug therapy before each prescription is dispensed.

Medicaid buy-in   A health care reform approach which would permit uninsured individuals to enroll in Medicaid by paying premiums on a sliding scale.

Medi-Cal   Medicaid in California. Since each state administers Medicaid, the program in California is unique (as are the programs in the other states).

medical   When applied as an adjective as in "medical treatment", this term means "nonsurgical," that is, the avoidance of the surgical methods of operation and manipulation. Synonym(s): nonsurgical.

Medical Assistance   See *Medicaid*.

medical association   See *medical society*.

medical audit (MA)   See *patient care audit* under *audit*.

medical audit study (MAS)   The operational unit of a "medical audit." See *patient care audit* under *audit*.

medical care   Traditionally, care which was under the direction of a physician. For a time, "medical care" came to refer only to those portions of the care provided directly or personally by a physician, with the care given by other professionals (such as nursing care, rehabilitation, and the like) excluded, or at least semi-independent, from the definition of medical care. So the term "patient care" was introduced. For example, "evaluation of medical care" was replaced in most usage by "evaluation of patient care"; the latter term not only focusing on the patient, but also ensuring that all components of the care — not just what the physician does — are included. The usage has changed, however, with "managed care" in many situations replacing "patient care".

medical care evaluation   Usually refers to the patient care audit (medical audit), which is a retrospective review of the quality of care of a group of patients, ordinarily a group with the same diagnosis or therapy. See *patient care audit* under *audit*.

medical care evaluation study (MCES)   See *patient care audit* under *audit*.

medical care hotel   A hotel for patients who need certain hospital services, but who can live in hotel surroundings, that is, without round-the-clock nursing. This is not a hotel for the families of patients.

   hospital medical care hotel   A medical care hotel operated by a hospital.

medical center   An essentially undefined term which may refer to a single institution, but is usually taken to mean that there is more to the institution than merely a single hospital—perhaps several hospitals in a complex, or perhaps a wider range of facilities and services than an ordinary hospital is likely to offer. The term does not automatically imply that the institution is an academic center, nor is there any licensure requirement before the term may be used.

   academic medical center   A medical center which ordinarily consists of a university hospital and medical school, often along with other teaching hospitals, research organizations and their laboratories, outpatient clinics, libraries, and related facilities.

Medical Directive, The   See *advance directive*.

medical director (health care plan)   A physician who contracts with or is employed by a health care plan (or other managed care organization) to provide medical direction. Responsibilities will include review of authorizations for referrals and admissions, review of cases for quality and utilization issues, formulation of clinical policies, criteria, and standards, and so forth.

medical director (hospital)   A physician, usually employed by the hospital, who serves as the administrative head of the medical staff. "Medical director" tends to be the title for the chief of staff when that person is a paid hospital employee. The title may also be "vice president for medical affairs" or something similar. This term is discussed further under *chief of staff*.

Medical Group Management Association (MGMA)   The national association of business managers of medical group practices.

Medical Illness Severity Grouping System (MedisGroups)   A proprietary system for classifying (2) hospital patients by severity of illness using objective data specially abstracted from the patients' medical records (see *abstract* and *abstracting*). This classification is a contender for use in supplementing the Diagnosis Related Group (DRG) classification to allow for severity. It was developed by MediQual Systems, Inc.

medical indigence   The condition of being medically indigent. See *indigent*.

medical informatics   See *medical informatics* under *informatics*.

Medical Injury Compensation Reform Act (MICRA)   A California statute enacted in the mid-1970s which has been proposed as a model for malpractice reform. Its provisions include caps on noneconomic damages; elimination of joint and several liability, and instead hold defendants liable only in proportion to their degree of fault; offsets by awards from collateral sources; limits on statutes of limitations; and limits on attorney contingency fees.

medical IRA   See *individual health care account*.

Medical Literature Analysis and Retrieval System (MEDLARS)   A   computerized, online database of the United States National Library of Medicine (a federal governmental agency).

Medical Management Analysis (System) (MMA)   A proprietary system for carrying out occurrence screening; a method for detecting cases in which there was a possible quality problem. Its author is Joyce W. Craddick, MD, president of Medical Management Analysis Consulting and Education Services, Inc., of Auburn, California.

Medical Outcomes Study (MOS) Short-form General Health Survey   See   *Medical Outcomes Study (MOS) Short-form General Health Survey* under *quality of life scale*.

medical record   A file kept for each patient, maintained by the hospital (the physician also maintains a medical record in his own practice), which documents the patient's problems, diagnostic procedures, treatment, and outcome. Related documents, such as written consent for surgery and other procedures, are also included in the record. The Joint Commission on Accreditation of Healthcare Organizations (JCAHO) places great importance on the medical record in the accreditation process, and its Accreditation Manual for Hospitals (AMH) contains an extensive description of the desired and required contents of the medical record.

Ordinarily the record is kept on paper, but it is increasingly being kept in computer (electronic) media as computer-based patient records (CPR). Occasionally a hospital keeps a separate medical record for each hospitalization (hospital admission); the better practice is to use the "unit record system," that is, keep a "unit record" for each patient, with all records of the patient's successive hospitalizations in the patient's unit file.

The record itself is usually organized in either the "traditional" or "problem-oriented" method (see below). The medical record is also called the clinical record, the patient's chart, or simply the chart.

computer-based patient record (CPR)   In 1991 the National Academy of Science's (NAS) Institute of Medicine (IOM) published the result of its study of the computer-based patient record (CPR). It identified twelve key attributes for the CPR, involving the information it should contain and its organization: 1) Problem list and problem-orientation of the information; 2) Measures of health status and functional levels; 3) Documents clinical reasoning and rationale; 4) Longitudinal and with timely linkage to other records on the patient; 5) Confidentiality, privacy, and audit trails; 6) Continuous access for authorized users; 7) Supports simultaneous multiple user views into the CPR; 8) Supports timely access to local and remote information resources; 9) Facilitates clinical problem solving; 10) Supports direct data entry by physicians; 11) Supports practitioners in measuring and managing costs and improving quality; and 12) System has flexibility to support existing and evolving needs of each specialty. A recent study indicates that no CPR meets these requirements. The IOM study is *The Computer-based Patient Record: An Essential Technology for Health Care.*

The computer-based patient record (CPR) is under development by a number of individuals and organizations. The Computer-Based Patient Record Institute (CPRI) was formed to pursue and coordinate the efforts. Additional and updated information is available on CPRI's Internet web home page at http://www.CPRI.org.

online medical record (OMR)   A medical record kept in a computer, with constant instantaneous access via a computer terminal and sometimes with other forms of data entry, such as point-of-sale (POS) terminals for laboratory and other data.

problem-oriented medical record (POMR)   A medical record organized around the problems presented by the patient. (See the definition of problem.) The POMR is organized so that the reader can find out *why* the steps in investigation and management were done. In the traditionally organized medical record, the reader can only find out *what* was done. A common form of organization of the POMR is "SOAP": Subjective (complaints), Objective (observations, test results), Assessment, and Plan for each problem. The same principle is increasingly used for nursing information and that of other professionals in the medical record; that is, nursing and other information is recorded in connection with the problem(s) to which it pertains.

traditionally organized medical record   A medical record organized according to "presenting complaint," "history," "review of systems" (such as cardiovascular and respiratory), "physical examination," and the like. The traditional organization tells only "what was done", while the problem-oriented medical record (POMR) tells "why it was done". The nursing record is traditionally organized chronologically.

Medical Records Institute (MRI)   An independent organization promoting electronic health records as a part of a seamless, patient-centered information system. Provides educational programs and publications in the field. Internet: http://www.medrecinst.com.

medical review agency   An agency established under the prospective payment system (PPS) to carry out certain surveillance functions with respect to hospital and physician performance and detection of fraud.

medical savings account (MSA)   A proposed mechanism for helping an individual provide funds for health care. It would be a savings account set up for an individual under regulations and tax treatment similar to an individual retirement account (IRA). The cash in the account would be available to pay for deductibles, copayments, and services not provided by the holder's insurance. The individual owning the MSA could keep any money not spent for health care. The theory is that this incentive would reduce unnecessary utilization. At present, employer contributions to MSAs are considered taxable income to the individual, while employer contributions for health insurance are not taxable income. Sometimes called a medical IRA.

management service organization (MSO)   A central service, created by a hospital for its physicians, or by one or more medical groups, which provides administrative services such as insurance and other billing, scheduling of consultations, referrals, and hospitalizations, facilities, equipment, and personnel, and so forth. Only one staff, that of the MSO, needs to become expert in the requirements of the various insurance carriers, and a single computer system is used, with terminals in the physicians' offices. Also called "medical service organization".

medical service organization (MSO)   See *management service organization (MSO)*.

medical society   A term generally used with reference to a geographically defined association of physicians, for example, a city, county, state, or national medical society. Associations whose membership is made up of specialists (for example, surgeons) are usually called "specialty societies." The medical staff of a hospital is not a medical society. Synonym(s): medical association.

medical staff   An organization of a hospital's medical staff members formed to carry out two functions: (1) to provide the management structure through which the hospital policies which pertain to the medical staff members are carried out, with particular attention to the quality of care; and (2) to serve as the spokesperson for the physicians to the governing body. This organization is variously referred to as the "medical staff," the "organized medical staff," the "medical staff organization," or simply the "MSO."

medical staff activities   A term used to include both the rights and duties of medical staff members. The rights include, primarily, the right to vote in medical staff meetings. The duties include carrying out the functions which devolve on members under the medical staff bylaws (see *bylaws*), including committee membership and participation, and accepting the supervision and sanctions laid out in the bylaws. All medical staff members are governed by the medical staff bylaws, which contain some provisions which affect all classes of members, such as those dealing with professional and personal conduct and completion of medical records.

medical staff corporation   See *medical staff corporation* under *corporation*.

medical staff member   A physician or other licensed health care professional who is permitted to care for patients independently in the hospital. Each medical staff member must be formally appointed to the medical staff by the governing body, and be authorized by that body to treat patients, independently, in the hospital. This appointment to the medical staff must be based on the individual being licensed and meeting the hospital's own requirements. Members are granted specific privileges by the governing body, delineating what they are permitted to do within the hospital, and are subject to the medical staff bylaws and rules and regulations and to review under the hospital's quality management program. In addition, all members must be reappointed periodically, and their privileges reaffirmed.

Physician practitioners on the medical staff are usually authorized to admit patients. Nonphysician practitioners usually do not have admitting privileges. For a discussion of the procedures for appointing physicians and other professionals to the medical staff, see *credentialing*; for more detail regarding admitting and clinical privileges, see *privileges*.

Members of the medical staff are often erroneously referred to as "hospital staff" or merely "staff"; in fact, members are usually physicians in private or group practices. Generally, "hospital staff" refers to hospital employees, while "staff" alone is ambiguous unless taken in context.

medical underwriting   See *medical underwriting* under *underwriting*.

medically indigent   See *medically indigent* under *indigent*.

medically underserved area   A rural or urban area which does not have enough health care resources to meet the needs of its population. The term is defined in the Public Health Service Act and used to determine which areas have priority for assistance. A "physician shortage area," also a designation of the Public Health Service, is a medically underserved area which is particularly short of physicians.

medically underserved population   A population group which does not have enough health care resources to meet its needs. The group may reside in a medically underserved area, or may be a population group with certain attributes; for example, migrant workers, Native Americans, or prison inmates may constitute a medically underserved population. The term is defined in the Public Health Service Act and used to determine which areas have priority for assistance.

Medicare   The federal program which provides health care to persons 65 years of age and older and to others entitled to Social Security benefits. Medicare is administered at the federal level, as contrasted with Medicaid, which is administered by the states. Medicare was established in 1965 by amendment to the Social Security Act, the pertinent section of the amendment being "Title XVIII—Health Insurance for the Aged." For a discussion of how payments are determined under Medicare, see *Omnibus Budget Reconciliation Act of 1989 (OBRA 89)*. There are two parts to Medicare:

Medicare, Part A   The hospital care portion (Hospital Insurance Program (HI)) of Medicare. Individuals who (1) are age 65 and over and who qualify for the Social Security "Old Age, Survivors, Disability and Health Insurance Program" or who are entitled to railroad retirement benefits; (2) are under age 65 but have been eligible for disability for more than two years; or (3) qualify for the end stage renal disease (ESRD) program are automatically enrolled in Part A of Medicare. Synonym(s): Hospital Insurance Program (HI).

Medicare, Part B   The part of Medicare through which persons entitled to Medicare, Part A, the Hospital Insurance Program, may obtain assistance with payment for physicians' services. Individuals participate voluntarily through enrollment and the payment of a monthly fee.

"Medicare fraud and abuse rules"Medicare fraud and abuse rules   See   *fraud   and   abuse.*

Medicare Geographic Classification Review Board (MGCRB)   The board, advisory to the Health Care Financing Administration (HCFA), which reviews applications from hospitals for their classification into one of the three tiers of reimbursement levels available to hospitals under Medicare.

Medicare Insured Group (MIG)   An organizational concept allowing businesses or labor unions to distribute Medicare funds to retired employees. By targeting a specific group of retirees, it is hoped that costs can be lowered through the use of managed care.

Medicare SELECT   An experimental program in 15 states in which Medicare beneficiaries purchase a type of Medicare supplement insurance product which covers supplemental services, but only if they are provided by designated preferred providers. Medicare SELECT was made possible by federal legislation in 1990 (OBRA) which permitted the program to be tested for a period of 3 years beginning in 1992. The states chosen by the Health Care Financing Administration (HCFA) were Alabama, Arizona, California, Florida, Indiana, Kentucky, Michigan, Minnesota, Missouri, North Dakota, Ohio, Oregon, Texas, Washington, and Wisconsin. Michigan and Oregon were later replaced by Massachusetts and Illinois. By late 1994, about 450,000 (about 3%) of the eligible beneficiaries had signed up.

In July of 1995 the program was continued until 1997, and expanded to all 50 states. At that time the SELECT program will be reviewed, and will continue indefinitely unless Congress ends it.

Medicare supplement insurance   Insurance which may be purchased by an individual to add to the benefits provided that individual under Medicare itself. Intelligent purchase of such insurance was virtually impossible until 1992, when uniform benefit packages, which standardized benefits for Medicare supplement insurance, were mandated by the federal government. A total of 10 standard plans ("A" through "J") were specified. No insurance company can offer such insurance with benefits below the minimum, Plan A. If an insurance company wants to offer more elaborate benefits, each offering must conform with one of the other nine plans, Plans B through J. Synonym: MediGap insurance. See also *wraparound coverage* under *insurance coverage.*

Medicare Volume Performance Standards (MVPS)   A type of expenditure target which was one element of the physician payment reform introduced by the Omnibus Budget Reconciliation Act of 1989 (OBRA 89).

medicine (substance)   A substance administered to treat disease.

medicine (science)   The science and art of the diagnosis and treatment of disease and the maintenance of health.

medicine (nonsurgical)   A general method of treatment of disease by means other than surgical; that is to say, "medical treatment" is treatment without surgery (without operation or manipulation).

medicine (system)   A system of diagnosis, and particularly treatment, based upon a specific theory of disease and healing.

allopathy   A system of medicine based on the theory that successful therapy depends on creating a condition antagonistic to or incompatible with the condition to be treated. Thus drugs such as antibiotics are given to combat diseases caused by the organisms to which they are antagonistic. Allopathy is the predominant system in the United States, and its practitioners are Doctors of Medicine (MDs).

chiropractic   A system of medicine based on the theory that disease is caused by malfunction of the nerve system, and that normal function of the nerve system can be achieved by manipulation and other treatment of the structures of the body, primarily the spinal column. A practitioner is a chiropractor, Doctor of Chiropractic (DC).

homeopathy   A system of medicine based on the theory that diseases should be combatted (1) by giving drugs which, in healthy persons, can produce the same symptoms from which the patient is suffering, and (2) by giving these drugs in minute doses.

osteopathy   A system of medicine which emphasizes the theory that the body can make its own remedies, given normal structural relationships, environmental conditions, and nutrition. It differs from allopathy primarily in its greater attention to body mechanics and manipulative methods in diagnosis and therapy. Osteopathy is second to allopathy in number of practitioners in the United States. Osteopathic physicians are granted the Doctor of Osteopathy (DO) degree (note that an "OD" is not an "osteopathic doctor," but an optometrist, an "optometric doctor").

medigap insurance   See *Medicare supplement insurance.*

medisave   See *medical savings account* and *MedAccess plan.*

MEDLARS-on-line (MEDLINE)   A network linkage system between a number of United States medical libraries and the Medical Literature Analysis and Retrieval System (MEDLARS) of the National Library of Medicine.

member   See *enrollee.*

mental health   The state of being of the individual with respect to emotional, social, and behavioral maturity. Although the term is often used to mean "good mental health," mental health is a relative state, varying from time to time in the individual, with some people more mentally healthy than others.

merger   The formal union of two or more corporations (such as hospitals) into a single corporation. In a merger, one of the original corporations retains its identity and continues to exist, while the other corporations are merged into it and lose their former identities. A consolidation is similar to a merger, except that all of the corporations which unite cease to exist, and a new corporation is formed with its own new identity. In either case, the surviving or consolidated corporation acquires the assets and assumes the liabilities of the former corporations.

meta-analysis   A research method which entails taking several studies on a given topic and analyzing those studies together, thus making a large study out of them. The method is of relatively recent development, and much attention is being given to improving the methodology itself. The study resulting using meta-analysis is also called a "meta-analysis."

method   A technique or procedure for doing something. Compare with *modality*.

method effectiveness   When a treatment fails to achieve its intended results, the failure may be due to the method employed or its use. For example, a contraceptive failure may occur because the method was inadequate or because it really was not employed (used) or was employed improperly. Thus the "method effectiveness" or the "use effectiveness" of the contraceptive may have been at fault, and the failure may have been a "method failure" or a "use failure."

method failure   When a treatment fails to achieve its intended results, the failure may be due to the method employed or its use. For example, a contraceptive failure may occur because the method was inadequate or because it really was not employed (used) or was employed improperly. Thus the "method effectiveness" or the "use effectiveness" of the contraceptive may have been at fault, and the failure may have been a "method failure" or a "use failure."

method or process patent   A patent for a method or process, comparable to a patent for a product or device. Under current patent law (1995) it is possible for a medical or surgical method or process to be patented, and for the patent holder to require the payment of royalties for use of the method. A surgeon in Arizona, for example, holds a patent on a "stitchless" technique used in cataract surgery, and is seeking to collect royalties from more than 2,000 ophthalmologists using the procedure. Other procedures for which patents have been obtained include one for determining the gender of a fetus by ultrasound methods and using injections of vasodilators to treat male impotence. The American Medical Association (AMA) has taken a stand against the patenting practice, and federal legislation has been introduced (1995) to ban the practice.

MICRA   See *Medical Injury Compensation Reform Act*.

micro measures   In health care, refers to steps taken to improve the health care provided to individual patients, rather than the health care system. See *macro measures*.

microeconomics   The economic theory which pertains to forces which determine the decisions and actions of individuals, rather than of entire populations. The latter theory is called macroeconomics.

microregulation   Regulation of the health care of patients at the level of the individual institution, physician, and patient. Not only does microregulation interfere with the freedom of all three, but it also significantly increases administrative costs and paperwork, because of the oversight system required to monitor the "behavior" of the physician, patient, and institution.

mind-body medicine   A philosophy of medical practice in which the major focus is on the whole person rather than on a physiological system. Attention is given to patient empowerment, emotional connections, families, and cultural and language barriers. Patients are encouraged to use support groups, and are taught such techniques as meditation, yoga, stretching, nutrition, and relaxation exercises. An increasing number of hospitals are establishing Centers for Mind-Body Health.

Minnesota plan   In 1992 Minnesota enacted "HealthRight" legislation which is being closely watched in the health care reform discussions. The law (1) establishes a commission whose goal is at least a 10% decrease in the annual rate of increase in health care costs; (2) establishes a voluntary, state-subsidized insurance called MinnesotaCare which is available to low-income persons on a sliding scale proportional to income, with a maximum premium, and with state subsidy; (3) places reform regulations on insurance companies to prevent such practices as exclusion of pre-existing conditions and to provide portability of benefits and work toward standardization of rates across contracts; and (4) gives special attention to the unique problems of rural communities. The stipulation that physicians practicing within state-approved guidelines are given defense thereby in malpractice litigation is attracting considerable attention. Minnesotans point out that the law outlines a state's responsibility to provide a health care system rather than approaching the problem from the citizen's right to health care.

mission-critical   A system whose failure is likely to result in failure to accomplish a given task. For example, a space-heating control system is primarily mission-critical; its failure will result in a cold or overheated house. A water heating control system is safety-critical, since its failure may result in a burned person.

modality   A therapeutic (treatment) method employing electrical or physical (as contrasted with chemical or other) means. "Modality" is often used incorrectly as a synonym for method.

Model HMO Act   Regulatory guidelines issued in 1972 by the National Association of Insurance Commissioners, who along with the National Association of HMO Regulators now update the Model Act. The Act is used by many states to regulate their HMOs, ensuring the delivery of basic health care services according to the appropriate standards of care.

monosonistic   From monopsony, a market in which there is only one buyer, and that buyer exerts a disproportionate influence on the market; a special type of oligopsony, in which there are a few buyers with such influence.

morbidity Illness, injury, or other than normal health. This term is often used in describing a rate (a statistical term). One type of hospital morbidity rate, for example, is the postoperative infection rate; it is the number of patients with infections following surgery, expressed as a proportion of those undergoing surgery, within a given period of time.

comorbidity As used in the prospective payment system (PPS), a diagnosis present *before* hospitalization which is thought to extend the hospital stay at least one day for roughly 75 percent or more of the patients with a given principal diagnosis. The presence of a comorbidity is reported in the PPS by placing, as a secondary ICD-9-CM diagnosis code in the patient's bill, a condition defined by PPS as a comorbidity. See also *complication*.

compression of morbidity The situation which results if persons are healthy until later in life than at present, that is, if disability is postponed more than death, so that an individual's period of disability preceding death is shorter, and the older population is both "older and healthier." The converse could be called "expansion of morbidity," so that the population becomes "older and sicker." Which will occur is not known; guesses about this aspect of the aging of the population are critical in planning for long-term care.

mortality A term that applies to death. This term is usually used in the phrase "mortality rate," which means the number of patients who died expressed as a proportion of those at risk (same as death rate).

multidisciplinary Made up of individuals from different fields. In the hospital, a committee on patient care which has members who are physicians, nurses, and managers, for example, is a multidisciplinary committee.

multihospital system A term which technically pertains to two or more hospitals under a single governing body. In current usage, "multihospital system" also applies to a number of formal and informal arrangements among hospitals, varying from sharing of one or two services, through a variety of leasing, sponsoring, and contract-managing schemes, to full-blown single ownership of two or more facilities. Synonym(s): chain organization, hospital chain.

multipayer system A health care reform approach which uses a number of payers, usually both private and public. The German-style system is a multipayer system. See also *single-payer plan*.

municipal Pertaining to a governmental unit. While "municipal" is commonly used to refer to a local governmental unit, such as a city or town, it can also be used in a broad sense to refer to the internal affairs of a state, nation, or people.

N

National Association of Insurance Commissioners (NAIC) An organization of state insurance commissioners which works toward development of uniformity in insurance regulation. Model laws, regulations, and guidelines have been developed for insurance companies, prepaid managed care plans, and state legislatures. Other NAIC activities include maintaining market-based information systems, monitoring legislative activity, conducting research, and providing consumer information. It also offers an accreditation program.

National Commission to Prevent Infant Mortality (NCPIM) A Washington DC-based organization promoting "resource mothers," the U.S. name for the individuals who, in the United Kingdom, are called "health visitors." These persons guide mothers through child care and also through the health care system. An effort of NCPIM is the Resource Mothers Development Project (RMDP), which seeks to introduce resource mothers into every community to help needy pregnant women and their children. The duties of resource mothers would appear to be identical to those of public health nurses. NCPIM is sponsored by Nestle.

National Committee for Quality Assurance (NCQA) An independent, nonprofit organization which is an accrediting agency for managed care organizations whose membership includes health care quality experts, employers, labor union officials, and consumer representatives. Its accrediting standards address quality, credentialing, members rights and responsibilities, utilization, preventive health services, and clinical records.

National Community Care Network Demonstration Program A demonstration program of the Hospital Research and Educational Trust (HRET) of the American Hospital Association (AHA) under a grant from the W. K. Kellogg Foundation.

National Council of Community Hospitals (NCCH) An association of over 150 nonprofit community hospitals and health care systems, large and small, whose members provide more than 50,000 hospital beds nationwide and are located in 30 states. NCCH is dedicated to the survival and increasing efficiency of community hospitals, which deliver 80% of the hospital services provided to patients in the U.S. Many of these hospitals also conduct programs of professional education and research.

national health care An approach to health care reform in which the government pays for and delivers health care. Sometimes used (inaccurately) as a synonym for the Canadian-style system.

National Health Corps A federal program for providing medical, dental, and nursing services to rural areas of the United States.

national health expenditures (NHE)   An economic indicator to show what the United States spends on health care each year. It is usually expressed as a percentage of the gross domestic product (GDP). The NHE is the sum total of all health care expenditures, including physician and hospital services, drugs, home nursing care, eyeglasses, dental services, and so forth, as well as administrative costs, construction, and research. The NHE for 1993 was $940 billion, equal to about 14% of the GDP.

national health insurance   A federally established and operated system of health care financing encompassing all (or nearly all) citizens. Such a system, not in effect in the U.S., would provide uniform benefits to all and be paid for via taxes. Distinguish this from national health service, in which the government is not only the payer, as here, but also the provider. This term encompasses "socialized medicine".

national health service   An approach to health care reform in which the government actually *owns* the hospitals and employs the physicians, thereby becoming the provider of health services. This is distinguished from national health insurance, in which the government is the sole payer, but not provider. Synonym(s): nationalized health care.

National Health Service Corps (NHSC)   A federal program to provide financial assistance for persons who are preparing for health professions, and in return obligating them to serve in areas where there is a shortage of health care professionals. They are placed by the U.S. Public Health Service. Also known simply as "The Corps."

National Information Infrastructure (NII)   An initiative of the federal government begun in 1992 to enhance the application of computer technology and telecommunications in all sectors of the society. The initiative calls for a partnership between the government and the private sector in which the government helps with development efforts, but the private sector owns and operates the NII. It is planned that the NII will ultimately connect the nation's homes, businesses, schools, health care facilities and social service providers via an interactive telecommunications network. The administration reasons that by making information accessible when and where it's needed, workers will be more productive, resulting in a global competitive edge, an improved standard of living, and even improved quality of life. By way of example, the information used by the authors to write the definition of this particular term were obtained via the Internet, an already existing part of the NII vision. Certain key technologies still need significant development in order for the NII to meet its goals, including: computer image recognition, computer speech recognition and language translation, digital libraries, electronic commerce (money), electronic security/privacy, satellite data communications, software agents, video teleconferencing, wall-size flat screen displays, and wireless personal computers. The NII's use of these technologies in connection with public health is stated to have high priority, particularly given their potential to improve access to health care. See also *Internet* and *telemedicine*.

National Library of Medicine (NLM)   The United States National Library of Medicine in Washington, DC.

National Research and Education Network (NREN) A computer network to link scientists, scholars, students, government workers, and business people. It was established by the High Performance Computing Act of 1991.

nationalized health care See *national health service.*

nationalized health insurance See *national health insurance.*

natural death act Legislation governing procedures by which a competent person can execute an advance directive concerning the withholding or withdrawal of life-sustaining treatment, in case of incompetence. See also *right to die.*

NCCH See *National Council of Community Hospitals.*

NCQA See *National Committee for Quality Assurance.*

negative incentive See *disincentive.*

negligence The failure to exercise reasonable care. In addition to its ordinary meaning, negligence has a specific legal meaning; it is one kind of tort which results in legal liability. The tort of negligence requires a duty to exercise reasonable care; a failure to exercise such care; and an injury which was proximately caused by that failure. One may commit a careless act, but if no one is injured as a result, there is no "negligence" as far as legal liability is concerned.

professional negligence In the context of health care, professional negligence is the failure of a professional to exercise that degree of care and skill practiced by other professionals of similar skill and training (and, in some states, in the same geographic locality) under similar circumstances (see *standard of care (legal)*). Such lack of care alone, however, will not result in legal liability; there must be an injury to the patient, and the injury must have been caused by the negligent act.

negotiated fee schedule A fee schedule for paying physicians or other health care providers, determined through collective bargaining. Synonym(s): negotiated payment schedule.

neighborhood health center A facility, located where it will be easy for patients to go, which provides various services short of inpatient care.

neo-no-fault compensation See *patients' compensation* under *compensation.*

nethead A person who is highly knowledgeable about and active on the Internet ("The Net").

netiquette The etiquette of the Internet.

network accreditation See *Health Care Network Accreditation Program.*

network (computer) See *local area network (LAN)* , *wide area network (WAN)*, and *Internet.*

network (health care) A network is an entity that provides, or provides for, integrated health services to a defined population of individuals. A network offers comprehensive or specialty services and has a centralized structure that coordinates and integrates services provided by components and practitioners participating in the network. The term broadly covers a wide variety of arrangements, including health maintenance organizations (HMOs), preferred provider organizations (PPOs), vertically integrated hospital delivery systems, home care networks, behavioral health networks, and physician-hospital organizations (PHOs), or any group of providers or insurers who contract to provide health services.

The amorphousness of the "network" definition is demonstrated by this caution from the the *1995-96 AHA Guide*, which has for the first time a listing of "integrated health delivery networks." The *Guide* notes that "Networks are very fluid in their composition as goals evolve and partners change. Therefore, some of the networks included in this listing may have dissolved, reformed, or simply been renamed as this section was being produced for publication."

Examples of arrangements which might be classified as networks include:

A.   Individual practice associations (IPAs) in which physicians and/or other health professionals provide their services through the IPA to a given prepayment plan. This model has no direct integration of the physicians with the hospital; that link is provided by the prepayment plan.

B.   Medical service organizations (MSOs) in which the hospital provides a single point through which many physicians can have such tasks as their billings to various insurance companies and their scheduling handled. Only one staff needs to become expert in all the insurance policies; only one call can schedule consultations, referrals, hospitalizations.

C.   Contracts between individual physicians and hospitals.

D   Hospitals employing physicians.

E.   Hospitals contracting with physicians. The purchaser deals with the hospital. The hospital often pays the primary care physicians by capitation, and the specialists by fee-for-service.

F.   Health maintenance organizations (HMOs) which contract with both physicians and hospitals, and which offer prepayment contracts.

G.   "Foundations" in which the physicians and hospital(s) are members. The purchaser deals with the foundation, who may have a variety of arrangements with physicians and with hospitals.

H.   "Health systems" in which all physicians are employed by the system, which also operates the hospital. Thus the purchaser can simply deal with the system.

I.   "Care management organizations" which interpose a care manager between the patient and physician to administer the provision of services within the defined benefit package.

J.   "Fully integrated" arrangements, which offer prepayment plans with defined benefit packages, i.e., they offer insurance packages to employers and other purchasers. Such plans typically manage the care as well. The philosophy of both the benefit package construction and the care management will vary from plan to plan.

See also *integrated health delivery network (IHDN)*.

networking   An informal relationship among individuals for exchange of information, counsel, and planning; a support group.

net worth   Assets minus liabilities; also called "equity."

NGT process   See *Nominal Group Technique*.

noetic Originating or existing in the intellect or the spiritual world. There are an increasing number of health care organizations which are emphasizing the integration of science and spirituality in order to enhance the "healing force," joining scientific medicine with a spiritual or noetic dimension, to create whole person and whole community health care.

no-fault See *no-fault compensation* under *compensation*.

nominal group A group "in name only." A type of group described by Delbecq, Van de Ven, and Gustafson in which individuals are together in the process known as the Nominal Group Technique (NGT).

Nominal Group Technique (NGT) A process developed by Delbecq, Van de Ven, and Gustafson for "increasing the creative productivity of group action, facilitating group decisions...and saving human effort and energy..." A nominal group is a group "in name only," a type of group in which individuals are together but do not talk or interact until late in the NGT process.

nonexempt distinct part unit A term used in Medicare, apparently to mean a part of the hospital considered by Medicare to qualify for a different pay rate than another part. For transfer in or transfer out purposes, Medicare considers a nonexempt distinct part equivalent to another hospital.

nonfederal Not owned or operated by the federal government.

nonprofit An entity whose profits (excess of income over expenses) are used for its own purposes rather than returned to its members (shareholders, investors, owners) as dividends. To qualify for tax exemption, no portion of the profits of the entity may "inure" to the benefit of an individual. See *inurement*. "Nonprofit" does not necessarily mean "tax-exempt"; see *tax exempt* and *501(c)(3)*. Also see *nonprofit corporation* under *corporation*, and *nonprofit hospital* under *hospital*. Distinguished from " for-profit."

nonsurgical See *medical*.

nonviable (cannot live) Not capable of living, as a baby born below a certain birth weight.

nonviable (cannot succeed) Not capable of being carried out or of succeeding, for example, "nonviable plans."

nosocomial Originating in a hospital. The term is sometimes confused with "iatrogenic," which refers to a disease or injury resulting from a diagnostic procedure, therapy, or other element of health care.

nuclear medicine The use of radioisotopes (radioactive forms of chemical elements) to diagnose and treat patients and for investigation. Some applications provide imaging ("pictures" of body structures and functions), while others provide diagnostic tests and treatment for diseases.

nurse practitioner See *nurse practitioner* under *practitioner*.

nursing differential   An allowance originally added to payments for Medicare patients in recognition of the greater cost of providing nursing services to elderly patients.

nursing home   An institution which provides continuous nursing and other services to patients who are not acutely ill, but who need nursing and personal services as inpatients. A nursing home has permanent facilities and an organized professional staff.

nursing service administrator   A registered nurse (RN) responsible for the overall administration and management of nursing services in a hospital. It is the highest nursing position in the hospital. The nursing service administrator may have the title "vice-president for nursing" or some similar title. The former title was "nursing director." Synonym(s): nursing director, nursing service director, chief of nursing.

nursing services   Those services normally provided by nurses, including personal care, administration of drugs and other medications and treatments, assessment of patients' needs and care requirements, and preparation of care plans for individual patients. Nurse practice acts (laws) in the various states place limitations on the tasks (for example, administration of intravenous medication) which can be performed by registered nurses (RNs), licensed practical nurses (LPNs), and allied personnel, with and without supervision.

nurturing   The provision of nourishment. In health care, the nourishment under consideration is that required for the mental, spiritual, emotional, and social well-being of the patient and family as well as their physical well-being. The topic is getting increasing attention as hospital stays are becoming shorter and hospitalization is often being avoided altogether; the nurturing formerly provided by the hospital is proportionately reduced. The situation is compounded in today's society by many factors, including family members' diminished acceptance of responsibility for nurturing one another. Health care organizations, community and church support groups, and others are increasing their efforts to assist with nurturing in the home and other settings.

nutriceutical   Nutrients which are alleged or proven to be active in preventing or treating disease. Vitamins, minerals, herbal remedies, and other supplements are the major classes of such products. Examples, with some of the claims made for them, are beta-carotene (prevention of cancer); fish oils, niacin, oat bran (prevention of heart disease); fiber-based appetite suppressants (weight control); garlic (for cholesterol reduction), and calcium supplements (prevention or treatment of osteoporosis). A large sale of these products occurs in "nutrition stores," rather than pharmacies. For many of them, the benefits are not proven, most of them cannot be patented, and to qualify them so that they could be sold as over-the-counter (OTC) drugs would require that their promoters provide substantiated statements on their benefits and risks.

nutrition   A field of science dealing with the relationships of food products and eating patterns to the development, growth, maintenance, and repair of living organisms.

nutrition assessment   Determining the nutritional status of an individual or a group through physical, biochemical, or dietary intake indicators.

O

OBRA 89   See *Omnibus Budget Reconciliation Act of 1989.*

occasion of service   A specific act of service provided a patient, such as a test or procedure.

occupancy rate   See *occupancy rate* under *rate (ratio).*

occupational health   An area of specialization in health care which concerns the factors (such as working conditions and exposure to hazardous materials) in an occupation that influence the health of workers in that occupation, and which is concerned generally with the prevention of disease and injury and the maintenance of fitness (because these factors are important in maintaining a stable work force).

Occupational Safety and Health Administration (OSHA)   A federal agency responsible for developing and enforcing regulations regarding safety and health among workers in the United States.

occupational therapy (OT)   Treatment by means of "occupational" activities, that is, tasks which are constructive and often will permit gainful employment. Occupational therapy is used primarily with disabled individuals, but is also used in retraining individuals after illnesses and accidents.

office audit system   A technique reported from Canada in which a review team goes into the offices of physicians whose practice is outside the hospital, and examines patient records (medical records) for the purpose of determining the quality of care.

Office of Health Technology Assessment (OHTA)   One component of the Agency for Health Care Policy and Research (AHCPR) of the Public Health Service (PHS), Department of Health and Human Services (DHHS). OHTA evaluates, on request from the Health Care Financing Administration (HCFA), the risks, benefits, and clinical effectiveness of new or unestablished medical technologies that are being considered for coverage under Medicare. The assessments of OHTA form the basis for recommendations to HCFA as to coverage policy decisions under Medicare. "Health Technology Assessment Reports" are produced from the data collected and analyzed by OHTA. The reports are available without charge from the National Technical Information Service (NTIS).

Office of Management and Budget (OMB)   The agency in the federal executive branch which prepares and monitors the budget.

Office of Technology Assessment (OTA)   A Congressional investigative body whose duties have to do with assessing the merits and applications of technology.

OLAP   See *Online Analytical Processing (OLAP).*

oligopsony   A market in which there are only a few buyers who exert great influence on the market. A special case of oligopsony is a monopsony, in which there is only one buyer.

OLTP   Online Transaction Processing. See *Online Analytical Processing (OLAP)*.

Omnibus Budget Reconciliation Act of 1989 (OBRA 89)   A federal act which, among other things, called for significant physician payment reform and increased funding for effectiveness research. The act amended Title XVIII of the Social Security Act by adding section 1848, "Payment for Physician Services". Among other things, section 1848 dealt with creating a fee schedule for the payment of provider services, the rate of increases in Medicare expenditures, and limits on the amounts that non-participating providers can charge Medicare beneficiaries. The establishment of the fee schedule replaced the "reasonable charge system" used to pay Medicare fees until January 1, 1992. OBRA 89 required that payments under the new fee schedule be based on nationally uniform "relative value units" (RVUs) which are related to the resources used in providing the service. Section 1848(c) of OBRA 89 established RVUs for physician work, practice (overhead) expense, and malpractice (liability insurance) costs. To account for geographical differences in the cost of providing services (rent is higher in New York City than in Saint Paul), the act implemented "geographical practice cost indices" (GPCIs), sometimes called geographic adjustment factors (GAFs). Each state is divided into one or more geographical regions and assigned a work, practice, and malpractice GPCI value for each region. Each RVU value is then adjusted by its corresponding GPCI value, resulting in a resource based relative value (RBRVU). When this number is multiplied by a federally determined "converter", the result is the actual dollar amount the provider is paid for providing the service to the Medicare patient. The converter, called a "conversion factor" (CF) by the feds, is different for surgical services, non-surgical services, anesthesia, and (beginning fiscal 1994) primary care services.

online   Electronically available from a local or remote location; can be accessed by computer with a modem or through a network. Often written as "on-line".

Online Analytical Processing (OLAP)   Computer software which uses *multi-dimensional* databases and thus provides more detailed analyses and greater analytical speed than formerly possible. OLAP is distinguished from "Online Transaction Processing (OLTP)", which typically uses relational databases which are characterized as being *two-dimensional* (rows and columns). OLTP software supports many users who are adding, editing, and removing individual records in a database, one record at a time. To do a query in this context involves searching many individual records, which could bring even a powerful computer to a standstill if it involved many millions of records. OLAP, on the other hand, tends to deal with data which is already summarized in such a way as to support what is known as "multidimensional data analysis". By pre-digesting or "consolidating" the values contained in many separate records and storing the results back into the database, there is now a third dimension (time, or "trend") to the database that allows a much faster response time, now matter how large the database has become. While the standard database language for two-dimensional, relational databases is Structured Query Language (SQL), OLAP databases will require a new language, possibly called MDSQL, for multi-dimensional structured query language.

online medical record (OMR)

online medical record (OMR)   See *online medical record (OMR)* under *medical record.*

On Lok   Short for On Lok Senior Health Services, a program in San Francisco's Chinatown which enables severely disabled and frail older persons to remain at home rather than be placed in nursing homes. (On Lok means "happy home.")

open access   See *managed care.*

open enrollment   An limited time period, usually occurring annually, during which individuals are given the opportunity to enroll in a health care insurance plan without medical screening, and without regard to their health status. Open enrollment is a characteristic of some Blue Cross and Blue Shield plans and some health maintenance organizations (HMOs). The time period is limited in order to minimize the potential for adverse selection. Open enrollment is an effort to approach community rating (see *rating*).

operating statement   See *income and expense statement.*

operation   Sometimes an operation is defined as identical with a "surgical procedure." In general usage, however, the term "operation" is rarely used for a single procedure; the term suggests an event of sufficient magnitude that it requires special preparation of the patient, use of an operating room, assistance to the operator by nurses and often other surgeons, sometimes anesthesia, and postoperative care. The term "procedure," on the other hand, usually refers to something which is discrete, and for which a relatively short time is required for execution.   An operation often actually consists of a number of procedures, and the array of procedures which make up a given operation will vary from patient to patient. For example, cholecystectomy (gall bladder removal) for one patient may include "exploration of the common bile duct," while for another, this procedure may be omitted. For this reason, a proper description of an operation requires that its procedures be listed.

optimal coding   Submission of a patient's bill with diagnosis and operation coding which will qualify for the highest reimbursement possible, yet avoid any suggestion to the payer's audit system that an attempt is being made to obtain unjustified reimbursement, i.e., to avoid interpretation of the bill as "overcoded". Computer systems which are intended to achieve optimal coding are commercially available to health care providers. Compare to under-coding and over-coding.

Oregon plan   In 1989 Oregon passed the Oregon Basic Health Services Act designed to insure that all citizens would receive at least basic health care. One part would expand Medicaid coverage to all residents below the federal poverty level. This would be done by prioritizing services to be offered on the basis of cost-effectiveness, and only offering those given higher priority (the top 587 out of 709 services ranked). A second part of the plan would require employers to cover employees and their dependents. A third would require the small insurance market to form an all-payers' high risk insurance pool.At the time of enactment of the law, Medicaid in Oregon was only able to cover 58% of the population below the federal poverty level; the goal is to cover 100% of this population, even though coverage will be more "basic." In 1991 the Oregon Department of Human Resources submitted to the Health Care Financing Administration (HCFA) a proposal to implement the resulting plan as a 5-year demonstration project to begin in January 1992.

organ procurement agency (OPA)   An agency set up to keep records of persons needing organ transplants and donor organs available, and to match the two with such speed that the surgery can be performed. Also, an organization designated by the Health Care Financing Administration (HCFA) as qualified to obtain and supply organs for transplantation in the Medicare program.

organizational liability   See *enterprise liability* under *liability (legal)*.

osteopathy   See *osteopathy* under *medicine (system)*.

out-of-area   Beyond the geographical service area of a managed care plan. Out-of-area medical care requires providers who are not participating with the plan. Thus, it is not ordinarily covered by the plan unless it is emergency or urgent care.

out-of-area insurance   See *out-of-area insurance* under *insurance*.

out-of-network   An adjective applied to a provider or a service when the provider is not a part of the health care network (or system) or the service is not available within the network, and thus the cost has not been the subject of prior agreement. May also be called "out-of-plan." The antonym is, of course, "in-network."

out-of-plan   See *out-of-network*.

out-of-pocket cap   See *out-of-pocket cap* under *cap*.

outcomes research   Research attempting to evaluate the relative benefits of various kinds of treatment and medical care by measuring the outcomes of the care. The basic question asked is "Does Treatment A or Treatment B give the better outcome?" This is, of course, followed by "How much better is the one than the other?" and "How costly is the treatment with the better outcome?" And finally, there follows an evaluation of the cost/benefit relationship.

outlier   A patient who requires an unusually long stay or whose stay generates unusually great cost. The term is used in the prospective payment system (PPS). About five or six percent of the budgets for regional and national rates have been set aside for payments for outliers. Outliers provide an escape hatch for the hospital, because they allow the hospital to negotiate for a fee higher than the Diagnosis Related Group (DRG) price which would otherwise apply to the patient. Outliers are of two kinds:

cost outlier   An unusually costly case.

day outlier   See *stay outlier*.

stay outlier   An unusually long stay. Also called day outlier.

outpatient (OP)   A person who receives care without taking up lodging in a care institution.

outpatient bundling   See *outpatient bundling* under *bundling*.

over-coding   Submission of a patient's bill with diagnosis or operation coding which suggests to the payer's audit system that an attempt is being made to obtain a higher reimbursement than was probably justified. An audit of the coding and billing is likely to be triggered by such coding. Computer systems which are intended to prevent this are commercially available to health care providers. Compare to under-coding and optimal coding.

P

pain management program   A specialized medical program for the management of chronic (and sometimes acute) pain, employing a multidisciplinary approach with medical, nursing, and allied health professionals. The national cost of treating pain is said to rank as the third highest health care cost, led only by cancer and heart disease.

palliative care   Treatment to relieve or reduce pain, discomfort, or other symptoms of disease, but not to cure. See also *comfort care*.

panel   A group of individuals, given a specific task. The term is used for groups such as the physicians who form a preferred provider organization (PPO), those who are convened to review a grant application, or in law, a group of people given the duty to review information, receive evidence, and make a decision.

pretrial screening panel   In malpractice cases, a group of physicians who review the case before trial and make a recommendation as to whether there was malpractice, and if so, the dollar amount of damages the plaintiff suffered as a result of it. The purpose is to encourage settlement; if one party turns down a settlement based on the recommendation, that party may be penalized if she loses at trial.

paradigm   One's view of "the way things are"; an implicit framework within which "everything" fits or is understood. In science, for example, one's "world view" restricts what problems are considered legitimate for study and what methods are acceptable to pursue them. Sir Isaac Newton's "laws" of gravity and motion, developed in the 17th and 18th century, governed much of the scientific thought for nearly two centuries. Einstein's paradigm not only explained the same phenomena, but also opened the way for new thought. When people thought the earth was flat, this paradigm governed thinking about stars, oceans, and travel. Proof that the earth was a sphere released entirely new thinking. See *paradigm shift*.

paradigm shift   The change in one's "world view" in moving from one paradigm to another: replacing an old paradigm with a new one. Such a change may take a lot of energy, and usually has far-reaching consequences.

Among the paradigm shifts emerging today in health are: (1) from the view that knowledge processing is limited to the human mind, plus "paper and pencil," to the view that knowledge processing can be successfully extended through use of computer technology; (2) from the view that the physician should assume a "paternal" role of caring and making decisions for the patient, to the view that empowered patients are competent to collaborate in their own health care and that, in fact, many wish to and can *direct* their own care; (3) from the view that the government is responsible for the health of the community, to the view that the community itself is responsible; and (4) from the view that health care providers are there to provide "health care," to the view that "health" rather than "health care" is their goal.

parameter   Any defining or characteristic factor, especially one which can be measured or quantified.

practice parameter   A parameter relating to clinical practice.   See *clinical practice guidelines* under *guidelines*.

parens patriae   "Parent of his country." A legal term referring to the power of the state to protect its people—specifically, those unable to care for themselves, such as minors (children) and the mentally incompetent.

Pareto principle   A principle which states that in any series of steps in a process, such as the diagnosis of a patient's problem, there are a "vital few" steps and a "trivial many." The procedure for identifying the vital few and the trivial many is called a Pareto analysis. The Pareto analysis makes feasible productive efforts at quality improvement since, once the "vital few" steps where efforts pay off can be identified, appropriate action can be taken. The Pareto principle is also the key to optimizing the care possible under a condition of limited resources. The principle was developed by J.M. Juran, an authority on quality, and named after an Italian economist named Pareto.

partnership   Two or more people (or organizations) carrying on a business for profit (for the purpose of making money). The law recognizes such an enterprise as a legal partnership, whether or not the partners have a verbal or written partnership agreement. In a general partnership, the partners share profits, losses, and management of the business, and are all equally liable should the partnership be sued. In a limited partnership, there is at least one general partner who manages the business, and one or more limited partners who put in money and share profits and losses, but who are liable only to the extent of their investments, and who do not have management control. To be recognized as a limited partnership, however, the business must comply with legal formalities.

passive smoking   See *involuntary smoking*.

patient   A person who has established a contractual relationship with a health care provider for that provider to care for that person. A patient may or may not be ill or injured. A patient who is ill or injured, or who otherwise presents a health problem, is often referred to as a "case."

patient advocacy   An allied health field developed to help patients with their complaints and problems in relation to medical care and hospital and other health care services, and with the protection of their rights. The practitioner may be called a patient advocate, a patient representative, a health advocate, or an ombudsperson. See also *health advocacy*.

patient card   See *smart card.*

patient care management   The determination of processes and procedures (such as diagnostic testing, administration of drugs, surgery, nursing, physical therapy, and others), their scheduling, and arranging for them in the care of the individual patient.

patient care manager (PCM)   Synonym for *gatekeeper.* It has been suggested that the term "PCM" replace the widely-used term "gatekeeper," but "gatekeeper" is likely to be retained.

patient-centered care   Health care which takes into account the patient's preferences, values, life style, family, expressed needs and fears; care approached from the patient's point of view. Such care includes education, physical comfort, emotional support, coordination of care, involvement of family and friends, and help with transitions.

patient days   The total number of inpatient service days, for all patients, during a specified period of time (for example, a month). Ordinarily this number will be expressed in three segments—adult days, pediatric days, and newborn days—since there almost certainly will be a desire to relate the usage in these three segments to the "adult inpatient bed count," the "newborn bed count," and the "pediatric inpatient bed count." Each bed count multiplied by the number of days in the period gives the "available bed days," the denominator in computing the occupancy rate.

patient-directed care   Health care guided by the recipient of the care. A trend in medical practice stemming from the concept that patients should be empowered to make decisions as to their own health and health care. In patient-directed care, the physician advises and collaborates with the patient in determining the steps to be taken to discover the causes of problems and in treating those problems. See *patient empowerment.*

patient dumping   See *dumping.*

patient education   See *patient education* under *education.*

patient empowerment   Enabling individuals to control their own health and health care decisions. "Empowerment" means granting power or authority; it also means enablement. Granting authority may mean simply giving permission, but enablement may also require the provision of information not ordinarily available and/or additional education. "Patient empowerment" requires using empowerment in both senses.

Patients have been given legal power at both the state and federal level. Many states have enacted a Patient's Bill of Rights, providing patients with both consumer and health care protections. The federal Patient Self-Determination Act supports the implementation of an individual's right to make decisions concerning extraordinary treatment.

Enabling individuals to make intelligent, informed decisions concerning their health care, however, involves more than merely giving them the "right." They need tools—mostly information—and the cooperation and assistance of their health care professionals. Patient empowerment requires a relationship between patient and physician (or other caregiver) in which both patient and physician understand that the patient has the authority to make (or share substantially in) the decisions concerning his or her medical care, with regard to both the diagnostic efforts to be employed and the treatment to be given. This collaborative relationship between patient and physician is called one of "shared decision making (SDM)".

Many physicians have become convinced that SDM is desirable — the care is based on the patient's values; patients comply better with the care process when they understand it and have helped select it; most patients are pleased to be treated as responsible individuals; and the outcome is often superior. But employment of SDM has been slow, in large part because of the "knowledge asymmetry" between the patient and the physician; that is, the professional knows a great deal more about medicine than does the patient. This problem is diminishing with the development of decision support software (DSS) systems, which provide current biomedical knowledge to guide both the physician and the patient at the time that the decisions need to be made. With these tools, the patient can become thoroughly informed as to the nature of the various options available, and their risks and benefits. The patient can then make truly informed decisions and can give truly informed consent.

Patient Outcomes Research Team (PORT) A research group supported by the Agency for Health Care Policy and Research (AHCPR) to conduct a specific study on a topic such as the values of various options for the treatment of prostate cancer and benign prostatic hyperplasia (BPH), the use of serum prostatic specific antigen (PSA) in screening for prostatic cancer, values of knee replacement surgery, and the treatment of back pain. PORTs were established in 1990 as a part of AHCPR's Medical Treatment Effectiveness Program (MEDTEP).

Patient Self-Determination Act (PSDA) A federal law which requires most hospitals, nursing homes, and other patient care institutions to ask all admitted patients whether they have made advance directives as to their wishes concerning the use of medical interventions for themselves in case of the loss of their own decision-making capacity. The institution is required to furnish each patient with written information about advance directives.

Patient's Bill of Rights A statement adopted by the American Hospital Association (AHA) in 1973 giving some 12 "rights" to which it felt that hospital patients were entitled. These include the right of the patient to be included in making treatment decisions, to be treated with dignity, to have privacy, and so forth. In several states, legislation has been passed codifying and augmenting these rights; some states extend these rights to nonhospitalized patients.

patients' compensation See *patients' compensation* under *compensation*.

payer An organization or person who furnishes the money to pay for the provision of health care services. A payer may be the government (for example, Medicare), a nonprofit organization (such as Blue Cross/Blue Shield (BC/BS)), commercial insurance , or some other entity. In common usage, "payer" most often means "third party payer".

fourth party payer See *fourth party*.

third party payer   A payer who neither receives nor gives the care (the patient and the provider are the first two parties). The third party payer is usually an insurance company, a prepayment plan, or a government agency. Organizations which are self-insured are also considered third parties.

payment   The act of paying or the amount paid for health care services.

peer review   Review by individuals from the same discipline and with essentially equal qualifications (peers). "Peer review" usually means review of the performance of a physician, done by other physicians, although it applies to such activity within any discipline. Peer review sometimes leads to reduction or denial of privileges of a physician (or other professional) whose performance is reviewed. It is therefore especially important that the process be done fairly and in good faith to avoid legal liability.

"Peer review" sometimes has a narrower meaning, which can be determined only after careful listening and asking: (1) some use the term only for review conducted by a group of physicians appointed by a medical society; (2) some use it as a synonym for a patient care audit; and (3) some use it only when the reviewers are physicians.   The term is also used in connection with review of research projects funded by the National Institutes of Health (NIH).

peer review committee   A committee of physicians, charged with review of the performance of other physicians.   The committee may be that of a medical society, hospital department, medical staff, or other entity.

Peer Review Organization (PRO)   An organization set up as a part of the prospective payment system (PPS) to carry out certain review functions under contract from the Health Care Financing Administration (HCFA).   PROs are external to the hospital; some were formerly Professional Standards Review Organizations (PSROs) and the functions of PROs are similar to those performed by PSROs.

The duties of the PRO include, for example: determining whether the medical records of Medicare patients support the diagnoses and procedures stated in the claims submitted; determining whether a changing pattern of care in a hospital, as reflected in its claims submitted, represents an actual change in the kinds of patients or their treatment, or is a fictitious result of the claims submission and reporting system; reviewing the medical necessity of DRG outliers; reviewing cardiac pacemaker implantations; and attempting to achieve certain changes in performance in hospitals within the jurisdiction of the PRO. A PRO is not the same as a hospital or medical society peer review committee.

Pepper Commission   An advisory body which in 1990 made recommendations as to universal health insurance coverage for both acute care and long term care, and recommended the play or pay method of financing (see *mandate*). Most of the members of the Commission were congressional leaders. The official name of the Commission was the U.S. Bipartisan Commission on Comprehensive Health Reform.

percentile   The size or magnitude of that element, in a series of elements that are arranged in order of magnitude, whose location in the series is at the designated percentage of the way from the small end of the series to the large end. For example, the 50th percentile is the magnitude of the element that is 50 percent of the way through the series—namely, the magnitude of the middle element, if the series has an odd number of elements. (Thus the 50th percentile is the same as the median).

Algorithms (sets of rules) for calculating percentiles vary, and so their results for a given series may also vary somewhat. This is because the concept of "percentile" is not precise. The following example gives some results of one commonly used algorithm:

Grading of students is a familiar use of the percentile. All the test scores (either percentages or raw scores) are placed in order from lowest to highest. If there are 80 students in the class, the 40th test score (from either end) is the 50th percentile (also known as the median). The 60th test score (from the low end) is the 75th percentile, the 72nd (again from the low end) is the 90th percentile (90 percent of 80 students (scores) is 72).

per diem rate   See per *diem rate* under *rate (charge).*

performance data   Data which are developed from the activities of an individual or institution. Traditional hospital statistics such as admissions and discharges, lengths of stay, and mortality are performance data. More sophisticated performance data can be developed from ongoing information systems, such as those for billing and medical records. These can describe patterns of medical and surgical management of cases, adherence to critical clinical practice guidelines, use of generic versus proprietary medications and conformance to recommended medication schedules, and similar information. .

periodic interim payment (PIP)   A system of providing Medicare funds to providers on a regular basis. Periodic payments may be made monthly or semi-monthly to a hospital, home health agency, or skilled nursing facility in the Medicare program, based on the institution's estimated annual Medicare revenue. Adjustments are made later when actual revenue figures become available. Such a system of payment is also sometimes employed by other payers.

periodic payments   A payment arrangement which allows money due to be paid in installments, over time, instead of in a lump sum. The term is used in regard to settlements (or judgments) in malpractice cases, which allow the defendant to pay for the patient's health care and other needs as those expenses accrue, or to pay a fixed sum in even portions over a given number of years.

per member per month (PMPM)   Refers to the cost (or charge) for a health care premium for an individual for one month. At this writing, the cost PMPM is in the range of $100-150.

personal care services   Those services required to take care of the activities of daily living (ADL).

personal services   Usually, services which are provided simply because the recipient wants them, rather than because they are essential to her medical or other care. Examples include beauty parlor services, catered meals, and the like. Such services are not included in the benefits of a health care plan. See also *personal care services.*

pharmacoeconomics   The study of the cost-effectiveness of health-related interventions. The name has appeared because the initial attention is being given to drugs, but it appears that these evaluations will also include other health services, such as medical and surgical techniques and procedures, both diagnostic and therapeutic, and the use of technological tools. About 300 articles were published in 1990 on these topics, and in 1992 a magazine entitled *Pharmaco-Economics* appeared.

pharmacoepidemiology   The study of the use and effects of drugs in a given population. Investigators using the methods of this discipline provide information used by, among others, agencies concerned with the regulation of medicines.

PHS   See *Public Health Service.*

physical therapy (PT)   The use of physical means such as exercise, massage, light, cold, heat, and electricity, and mechanical devices in the prevention, diagnosis, and treatment of diseases, injuries, and other physical disorders. Physical therapy does not include the use of X-rays or other types of radiation. Synonym(s): physiotherapy.

physician   A person qualified by a doctor's degree in medicine (allopathy, homeopathy, or osteopathy). To practice, a physician must also be licensed by the state. Note that "physician" is the generic term; a surgeon is also a physician, but a physician is not necessarily a surgeon.

nonparticipating physician   Under Medicare, a physician who has not signed a contract agreeing to refrain from charging a Medicare patient the difference between the physician's usual charge and the Medicare payment allowance.

participating physician   Under Medicare, a physician who has signed a contract agreeing not to charge a Medicare patient for the balance between the physician's usual charge and the Medicare payment allowance for the service rendered.

primary care physician (PCP)   A physician who specializes in primary care (family practice, general internal medicine, general pediatrics, or obstetrics and gynecology). Provides the initial care for a patient, and refers the patient, when appropriate, for secondary (specialist) care.

referring physician   A physician who has asked another physician to give a consultation or to take over the care of a given patient, or who has sent a patient to another institution.

secondary care physician (SCP)   A specialist; one who treats patients on referral from another physician, most often a primary care physician.

physician contingency reserve (PCR)   See *withhold.*

physician extender   An allied health professional (AHP) who, under the supervision of a physician, provides services formerly given by physicians themselves. Nurse practitioners, advanced practice nurses (APN), midwives, and physician assistants are among those AHPs who serve as physician extenders.

physician-hospital organization (PHO) A legal entity formed by a hospital and a group of physicians. The PHO serves as a negotiating and contracting unit to obtain managed care contracts directly with employers. The physicians usually maintain their own practices, and contract with the PHO to provide services.

physician-hospital-community organization (PHCO) Same as a physician-hospital organization (PHO), except that the community is also represented on the governing board along with the hospital and physicians.

physician payment reform (PPR) A basic change in the way physicians were paid for services for Medicare patients, mandated by the Omnibus Budget Reconciliation Act of 1989 (OBRA 89), effective 1 January 1992. Prior to that date, payment had been based on customary, prevailing, reasonable charges (CPR). Replacing that method, the new method was based on a resource-based relative value scale (RBRVS). One intent of the change was to reduce the premium (high fees) put on procedures, typically done by specialists, and increase the reimbursement for cognitive services, such as evaluation and diagnosis and patient management, services provided mainly by primary care physicians. A second component of the reform was application of Medicare Volume Performance Standards (MVPS), targets against which physician's spending is measured. If a physician's standard is exceeded, the next year his or her rate of fee increase is reduced. A third component of the reform is a cap on the out-of-pocket charges which may be made to beneficiaries.

physician recruitment Finding, soliciting, and attracting physicians to a particular hospital or area. Hospitals devote resources to the search, and provide incentives, for physicians in specialties which are needed by the hospital and community. Such incentives may include relocation reimbursement and either initial employment of the physician or provision of a loan (with favorable terms) to enable the physician to start and build a practice in the area. Physician recruitment sometimes raises issues of inurement (private gain to an individual from the profits of a nonprofit corporation). For example, if the hospital pays the physician a salary in excess of reasonable compensation, or provides an interest-free loan, these incentives may be considered by the Internal Revenue Service (IRS) to be inurement and thus jeopardize the hospital's tax exempt status. The hospital must show that it (and the community) receive measurable value for the incentives provided.

physician shortage area A medically underserved area which is particularly short of physicians. The term is defined in the Public Health Service Act and used to determine which areas have priority for assistance.

physician's assistant (PA) A person who assists a physician by carrying out designated tasks, such as taking medical histories and performing certain examinations. May or may not be a trained allied health professional.

Physicians' Current Procedural Terminology (CPT, CPT-96, etc.) A publication of the American Medical Association (AMA), containing its classification of procedures and services, primarily those carried out by physicians. It is widely used for coding in billing and payment for physicians' services, including the Health Care Finance Administration's HCPCs. Each "package" of physician services (for example, care for a fracture—including diagnosis, setting the fracture, and putting on and removing the splint) is given one code number and commands one fee for the package. In contrast to *CPT*, ICD-9-CM, the classification used for hospital coding of diagnoses and procedures, has separate codes for each of the four factors: diagnosis, setting the fracture, applying the cast, and removing the cast.

CPT is similar in theory to the diagnosis related groups (DRGs) (which currently apply to hospital—not physician—care) in that both are built on the "one code, one fee" basis. Although the fourth edition of *CPT* appeared in 1977 (at which time it was called "CPT-4"), it has been revised repeatedly since then, and now the volume is labelled annually, for example "CPT-96". A CPT code can be recognized as a five digit number falling into the range of 00100 to 99499.

Physician's Payment Review Commission (PhysPRC)   A federal advisory body set up to provide input to the Health Care Financing Administration (HCFA) regarding methods of saving money in the payment of physicians for services to Medicare patients.

PKC   See *problem-knowledge coupler*.

Planetree   A consumer health care organization founded in 1978 as a nonprofit corporation. Its philosophy is based on consumer access to health and medical information, involvement of family and friends, and encouraging consumers to become active participants in improving, maintaining, and restoring their health. Planetree was created to humanize, personalize and de-mystify the health care system for patients and their families. Planetree assists health care providers in identifying and overcoming obstacles in delivering humanistic care. Some of the areas addressed by the organization are nursing, family involvement, patient education, and architectural design. Planetree has developed five Model Hospital sites in the United States, and about 20 affiliates in the United States and Europe as examples of this approach to patient-centered care. In addition it has implemented a nationwide Hospital Alliance with 18 members (1994) and has developed Health Resource Centers to give lay people easy access to health and medical information.

planning   The analysis of needs, demands, and resources, followed by the proposal of steps to meet the demands and needs by use of the current resources and obtaining other resources as necessary.

community-based planning   Planning in which the attempt is made to have the planning initiative in the local community rather than external to the community itself.

comprehensive health planning (CHP)   Attempts to coordinate environmental measures, health education, health care, and occupational and other health efforts to achieve the greatest results in a community.

health planning   Planning (a formal activity directed at determining goals, policies, and procedures) for a health care facility, a health program, a defined geographic area, or a population. Health planning may be carried out by the organization itself or by a planning agency. When it is carried out for an area, and the people in the area itself furnish the initiative, it is called "community-based planning."

joint planning   Planning carried out jointly by two or more institutions, which may or may not envision sharing of services and facilities..

strategic planning   A term derived from "strategy" in the military sense; planning which is long-range, and which is intended to lay out the nature and sequence of the steps to be taken to achieve the large goals of the organization. In traditional thinking, strategic planning should precede the development of the tactics with which it is implemented. A current insight is that a successful strategy can only be developed after the available tactics are assessed and used to their maximum.

play or else   See *employer mandate* under *mandate*.

play or pay   See *play or pay* and *employer mandate* under *mandate*.

plunge   An educational visit to an unfamiliar environment. The term is being used in health care for a visit to a community in order to begin to learn about its population, organizations, resources, problems, needs, and interests.

pluralistic system   A system which provides alternatives. The U.S. is described as favoring pluralism, as illustrated by the fact that medical care, for example, can be obtained from solo practitioners or group practices or prepaid health plans.

point-of-service (POS)   Selection of a provider by a managed care plan enrollee at the time (and *each* time) the care is needed. The entire plan may be designed as point-of-service, or the *option* may be offered to enrollees, usually for a higher premium and/or copay amount. Most managed care plans require the enrollee to use only in-plan physicians and other providers, except in emergencies or when out of the service area. With POS, the provider need not be a participant with the plan; an enrollee may select in-plan or out-of-plan providers. A plan not allowing the POS option is referred to a point-of-enrollment plan.
     Effective in October 1995, health care plans which accept Medicare risk contracts must offer each beneficiary a POS option under which the plan retains responsibility for the care provided, even though the service is not given by a provider who is under contract with the plan. POS plans are also known as "open-ended HMOs."

police power   The authority of government to restrict the rights of individuals to protect the health and welfare of the public. In the health care context, police power may be invoked by public health officials, for example, to quarantine infected individuals in order to control an epidemic, or to carry out an unannounced inspection of a restaurant, housing, or institution to ensure compliance with health and safety codes.

political action committee (PAC)   An organization which receives contributions, usually from individuals, and disburses them to candidates for office. May also engage in lobbying activities.

POMR   See *problem-oriented medical record* under *medical record*.

Ponte Vedra Group   An informal ad hoc "think tank" founded by John Horty, LLB, President of the National Council of Community Hospitals (NCCH), in 1992. Its first position on health care reform is that a single national solution to all the problems is not possible, that the movement already underway in which health care reform is emerging in local communities from the bottom up in response to those communities' specific needs and resources should be facilitated. Certain legislative changes which would encourage local innovation in health care organization and payment are encouraged, as are changes in favor of universal coverage and community rating for health insurance, tort reform, provision of portable benefits, and adoption of antitrust policies which would favor cooperation and collaboration among providers in order to preserve the patient care value system in the health care field.

In addition to these "macro" measures in health care reform, its second position is that every effort should be made to use the emerging technologies which make possible addressing specifically the problems of each individual patient, a "micro" approach to health care reform which promises improved quality for each person, and lowered cost for each encounter.

population medicine Health care in which the goal is the improvement of the health of a population, such as reduction in teen-age pregnancies, obesity, increase in cardiovascular fitness, in contrast with individual medicine which concerns the health of an individual.

portability An attribute of a health care payment system in which the beneficiary can move from one employer to another without loss of benefits or having to go through a waiting period. Without portable coverage, individuals often are unwilling to change employment because benefits will be lost. This condition is known as job lock.

positioning A term used in public relations (marketing) indicating the place occupied by an institution or product in the minds of its constituency. For example, IBM is "positioned" in the number one spot with respect to computers in most peoples' minds. Hertz has the same position in car rentals.

PPS See *prospective payment system* and *prospective pricing system.*

practice (action) To carry on a profession.

delegated practice The medical activities of nonphysician providers performed under the authority and direction of a licensed physician.

practice (business) A business in which a profession, such as medicine, is carried out.

group practice A medical practice consisting of three or more physicians or dentists, associated to share offices, expenses, and income.

multi-specialty group practice Group practice offering more than one medical specialty.

prepaid group practice Group practice providing care for a defined population under a prepayment arrangement.

single-specialty group practice Group practice in which all members of the group practice the same specialty.

solo practice A practice in which the physician (or other professional) is alone, that is, not a member of a group or associated with other physicians. Solo practitioners may, however, arrange with others to provide care for their patients in cases of the practitioner's absence or illness.

practice parameters See *clinical practice guidelines* under *guidelines*.

practitioner An individual entitled by training and experience to practice a profession. Often such practice requires licensure, and the boundaries of the practice are prescribed by law.

general practitioner (GP) A physician who does not hold specialty qualifications, and who does not restrict his practice to any particular field of medicine. Sometimes called a family practitioner. In recent years it has become possible for a physician to specialize in family medicine (become board certified in that specialty), and become a family practice (FP) specialist. General practitioners are primary care physicians.

independent practitioner An individual, usually a person who gives patient care, who practices without supervision. In a hospital, an independent practitioner must ordinarily be licensed and also must be granted specific privileges by the hospital.

nurse practitioner A registered nurse (RN) who has completed a nurse practitioner program at the masters degree or certificate level beyond basic nursing education. Nurse practitioners have qualifications which permit them to carry out expanded health care evaluation and decision-making regarding patient care. Nurse practitioners are, in turn, specialized into "family nurse practitioners," "gerontological nurse practitioners," "school nurse practitioners," and the like. The term "practitioner" implies a certain degree of independence from the supervision of a physician in making decisions and carrying out acts, with the boundaries of this independence stipulated by state law. Nurse practitioners are ordinarily regulated by state nurse practice acts.

preadmission certification (PAC) A process by which elective care which is proposed for a patient is reviewed and approved before the patient is admitted to the hospital. When a PAC program is in effect, the care will not be paid for unless the certification is obtained.

preadmission process for admission A formal admission process (namely, initiating the paperwork) carried out by a hospital prior to doing preadmission testing (PAT) for an elective admission patient.

preadmission screening (PAS) A program of evaluation of applicants for admission to nursing homes under Medicare. Some states also require preadmission screening for private pay applicants.

preadmission testing (PAT) The carrying out of laboratory and other diagnostic work on an outpatient basis within a few days of hospital admission for the patient scheduled for elective hospitalization. It is less costly to have the tests performed in this manner and, in some instances, the test results will be such that hospitalization will be avoided or postponed. The hospital usually goes through a formal acceptance of the patient, called the "preadmission process for admission," prior to carrying out the tests.

precautions Actions taken to prevent an undesired effect or outcome. In the health care context, "precautions" usually refers to measure taken to prevent the transmission of disease to a patient who is particularly vulnerable to infection because their immune system has broken down (such a patient is called a "compromised host"), or from a patient with an especially communicable disease. In the past, individual patients were designated as requiring special precautions, which were then taken only with respect to those patients. Gowns and gloves were worn in the patient's room, for example, and visitors were strictly limited. With the advent of AIDS, however, universal precautions have been instituted.

universal precautions (UP) A set of policies and procedures recommended by the Centers for Disease Control and Prevention (CDC), and required by the Occupational Safety and Health Administration (OSHA), for protecting patients, hospital staff, and physicians from the risk of contracting diseases, such as AIDS and hepatitis B, which are transmitted by blood and body fluids. "Universal" means that the precautions are to be taken with respect to *every* patient, not just those who are known to be particularly vulnerable or contagious. Recommended precautions include the use of gloves and special disposal of hypodermic needles to reduce accidental needlesticks.

predatory pricing A practice by insurers of giving a low rate on health insurance to a low-risk small group or individual, then raising the rates when the insured start filing claims. See also *cherry picking*. Synonym(s): churning the books, price churning.

preexisting condition A physical or mental condition which has been discovered before an individual applies for health insurance. Insurers often deny insurance to individuals with certain preexisting conditions, or invoke a waiting period, or reject a group unless such individuals are excluded. Health care reform efforts today insist that there be no exclusion of individuals for such conditions.

preferred provider arrangement (PPA) A form of organization for physician services, in a health care plan, in which the plan (the third party payer) establishes a roster of physicians who are believed to be cost-effective. All services covered by the plan, when furnished by these physicians, are without charge to the beneficiary. The beneficiary may elect care from physicians not on the roster, but if she does, at least part of those providers' fees must be paid by the beneficiary (or, in some forms of health insurance programs, by the physicians making up the roster of preferred providers).

preferred provider option (PPO) A form of health care plan in which certain physicians are designated by a third party payer as preferred providers whom the payer has concluded are the most cost-effective. When a beneficiary elects to receive care from these physicians, the physicians' charges are paid in full—there is no additional charge to the beneficiary. The beneficiary may elect to obtain care from other physicians, but if she does, there is a financial penalty to the beneficiary—she must pay part of the charges.

preferred provider organization (PPO) An alternative delivery system (ADS) designed to compete with health maintenance organizations (HMOs) and other delivery systems. A PPO is stated to be an arrangement involving a contract between health care providers (both professional and institutional), and organizations such as employers and third party administrators (TPAs), under which the PPO agrees to provide health care services to a defined population for predetermined fixed fees. PPOs are distinguished from HMOs and other similar organizations in that: (1) PPO physicians are paid on a fee-for-service basis, while in other delivery systems payment is usually by capitation or salary; and (2) PPO physicians are not at risk—the purchaser of the service retains the risk—while HMOs are at risk. The term "contract provider organization (CPO)" is preferred by the American Medical Association (AMA) for the arrangements discussed here. The term "CPO" might be preferable as a method of distinguishing a preferred provider organization from the other "PPO"—the preferred provider option. See also *exclusive provider organization (EPO)*.

premium A payment required for an insurance policy for a given period of time.

prenatal care Care for a pregnant woman in an effort to keep the woman healthy and to maximize the likelihood that the pregnancy will result in a full-term, full birth-weight, healthy infant.

prepaid health plan See *health care plan*.

prepayment plan A contractual arrangement for health care in which a prenegotiated payment is made in advance, covering a certain time period, and the provider agrees, for this payment, to furnish certain services to the beneficiary, member, or enrollee.

President's Task Force on National Health Care See *Task Force on National Health Reform*.

prevailing When used in conjunction with physicians' fees, "prevailing" refers to the charges made for the service in question in the area, provided by physicians of similar specialty qualifications.

prevalence The number of events or cases of disease present in a given population at a given time. "Prevalence" is often confused with "incidence," which is the number of new events taking place in a defined period of time in a specified area or population. Usually both incidence and prevalence refer to cases of disease or injury. Both are numerators in the calculation of an incidence rate or a prevalence rate, respectively, for the event in question. The denominator is, for both, the population at risk (the given population).

preventive health services Services designed to (1) prevent disease or injury from occurring, (2) detect it early, (3) minimize its progression, and/or (4) control resulting disability.

price   The amount of money to be paid for something. Each Diagnosis Related Group (DRG), for example, carries a price, the amount of money to be paid for the hospital care of a patient classified to that DRG.

price blending   A method of adjusting a hospital's price for a given Diagnosis Related Group (DRG) under the prospective payment system (PPS) after comparing the hospital's cost per case for that DRG with the national average for the same DRG. Synonym(s): DRG-specific price blending.

price-elasticity   A condition in which a seller can increase revenue by *reducing* prices (achieved, of course, by increased volume of sales). Under managed competition, price-elasticity is a specific goal. See *price-inelasticity*.

price-fixing   Two or more competitors agreeing on prices (charges). Price-fixing is a per se violation of the Sherman Act, an antitrust law.

price-inelasticity   A condition in which a seller can increase revenue by *raising* prices. Managed competition seeks to avoid price-inelasticity. See *price-elasticity*.

primary care   The care by a primary care physician (PCP). Care requiring more specialized knowledge or skill is obtained by referral from the primary care physician to a specialist (secondary care physician (SCP)) for consultation or continued care. The term is also used to mean the care given at the initial contact of the patient with the health care system or with a health care provider. It usually takes place in an office or other outpatient setting.

The definition proposed by the Institute of Medicine (IOM) in 1995 is: "Primary care is the provision of integrated, accessible health care services by clinicians who are accountable for addressing a large majority of personal health care needs, developing a sustained partnership with patients, and practicing in the context of family and community".

primary care center (PCC)   An institution for furnishing primary care. A PCC may be free-standing or part of another institution.

primary care network   A group of primary care physicians who have formed a network in order to share the risk of providing services to enrollees in a prepaid plan.

principal (legal)   A person (or entity, such as a corporation) who authorizes another to act on his or her behalf as an agent.

prion   A newly-identified class of infectious agents which consist of protein and nothing else, i.e., they do not contain genetic material (nucleic acid (DNA or RNA)), material previously thought necessary to establish an infection in a host. Prion diseases typically are fatal, destroying portions of the brain. They occur quite frequently in animals; examples are scrapie in sheep and goats, "mad cow disease" in Great Britain (more than 130,000 cattle since 1986). In humans, prions have been shown to cause "kuru" in New Guinea, Creutzfeldt-Jakob disease, Gerstmann-Straussler-Scheinker disease, and fatal familial insomnia. Pronounced "preeon", the word stems from small PROteinaceous INfectious particle.

privilege   A special right, benefit, or advantage granted to one person or a group or entity, but not to everyone.

privileged communication   Information which is legally protected from discovery in a lawsuit or use as evidence in a trial. Communications between a physician and patient are privileged communications, and cannot be revealed without the permission of the patient or a court order; most of the contents of a medical record are protected by this privilege. It should be noted that the privilege "belongs" to the person protected and can only be waived by that person; in this instance, the patient is the one whose rights are protected, so the privilege cannot be waived by the physician (or hospital), nor can the physician invoke the privilege if the patient waives it.

privileges   Rights granted by the governing body of the hospital to physicians and other health care professionals, who are members of the medical staff, giving them permission to carry out specified diagnostic and therapeutic procedures within the hospital and, in some cases, to admit patients. Privileges are granted upon recommendation of the medical staff, usually working through its credentials committee, which reviews the person's credentials and performance in determining the privileges to be recommended. Privileges may be withheld, increased, diminished, or withdrawn by the governing body at its discretion (subject, of course, to due process requirements). See also *credentialing* and *recredentialing*.

admitting privileges   Authority, granted by the governing body, to admit patients to the hospital. Generally, admitting privileges are restricted to physicians (MD and DO) and to podiatrists and qualified oral surgeons who are active members of the medical staff. The privileges ordinarily are limited with respect, for example, to the "kinds" of patients a physician may admit; a specialist in obstetrics and gynecology would not likely be granted privileges to admit psychiatric patients.

clinical privileges   Rights granted by the governing body of the hospital to a physician or other health care professional, who is a member of the medical staff, designating the types of diagnostic and therapeutic procedures the individual is permitted to perform, and also the types of patients that person is permitted to treat. Privileges granted are based upon the professional's education, training, and licensure, i.e., credentials, and on performance. "Other health care professionals" may include dentists, podiatrists, clinical psychologists, nurse practitioners, speech pathologists, physical therapists, and others, depending upon hospital policy as to requirements for membership in the medical staff.

Privileges are determined upon initial appointment to the medical staff, and are subject to formal review periodically (usually no less frequently than every two years, or more frequently if required by law), and also ad hoc upon the practitioner's request or on the basis of allegations of performance problems. Privileges are expanded as the physician (or other professional) acquires additional credentials and/or experience and demonstrates proficiency; they should be reduced if warranted by the physician's performance (subject, of course, to due process requirements).

Provisional privileges are granted initially, with performance being observed by peers (other physicians or peer professionals on the medical staff) and periodically reviewed with the assistance of hospital personnel who collect data and provide it to a review body (usually the medical staff member's clinical department) which makes recommendations to the credentials committee. Such periodic review continues for all medical staff members, even after the "provisional" requirements are dropped; it is a necessary part of quality management and of the process of reappointment of medical staff members. When used in the statement that a certain physician "has clinical privileges" in a given hospital, the term indicates that the physician has been granted membership in the medical staff of that hospital in a category which permits her or him to treat patients there.

prn   As (often as) or if necessary.

problem   A disease, injury, or any other condition or situation which brings an individual into contact with the health care system. Certain conditions, such as alcoholism, are not admitted by all to be diseases, but they do bring individuals to health care, as do ill-defined symptoms, behavioral problems, the need for well-person examinations, and the like. This is the usage of the term "problem" in the "problem-oriented medical record (POMR)".

Chapter XXI of the International Statistical Classification of Diseases and Related Health Problems (ICD-10), entitled "Factors Influencing Health Status and Contact with Health Services," lists among others the following "factors": loss of love relationship (code number Z61), removal from home (Z61), failed exams in school (Z55), stressful work schedule (Z56), and extreme poverty (Z59.5).

problem knowledge couplers (PKCouplers)   Interactive computer software for common PC computers which elicits (profiles) the significant attributes of a patient's problem and then matches (couples) this profile of the patient with the existing literature which has a bearing on the understanding of or solution to that problem.

The concept was conceived by Lawrence L. Weed, MD, who developed the problem-oriented medical record (POMR). The purpose of PKCouplers is to assist the physician and other providers in accessing the medical knowledge available in the literature as to diagnosis and management of patients, and to do it instantly on demand, while patient and physician are together. Four kinds of PKCouplers are available, (1) baseline, (2) diagnostic, (3) management, and (4) triage.

PKCouplers not only prove invaluable in coping with the information explosion in health care, but in providing the patient with knowledge — making the patient a true collaborator in reaching decisions about life style, diagnostic efforts to be expended, and treatments to be undertaken. Furthermore, couplers, computerized and cumulative, are important building blocks toward a computer-based medical record (CPR) which not only keeps a record, but also assists and guides the caregiver and patient.

baseline problem knowledge coupler   A class of PKCouplers which is typically used at the patient's first visit to provide a baseline of data about the patient. Under the heading of wellness, it collects information about the patient's life style, habits, and health risks. It also develops a thorough medical and health history, and records baseline physical and laboratory findings. If any of the inventories detect life style modifications or risk avoidance which would be beneficial, these are suggested to the physician and patient by the software. If medical problems are noted, the problem-specific diagnosis or management PKCouplers for them may be used to guide further investigation and management. Printouts are available for the patient and for the paper-based medical record.

diagnostic problem knowledge coupler   A class of PKCoupler which uses, as all PKCouplers, a two-step process. First it has a questionnaire which, when completed, constructs a patient's personal profile (database) for a given problem. This is done within a computer program which then, as step two, couples (matches) that profile with the medical literature's knowledge for the same problem.

The diagnostic PKCoupler for a given problem is structured to elicit data known to be helpful in discriminating among possible causes of the problem. Sources of the data are the patient's history, physical examination, investigative findings, response to therapy, and other factors. The knowledge database for that problem contains information on these same data items, maintained to reflect the current medical literature. Once the diagnostic coupler's patient profile is in the computer, where it is placed as a part of acquiring the data, coupling, on the physician's command, instantly matches the profile with the stored knowledge. The computer display (and printout) indicates which findings of the specific patient match each of the diagnoses (possible causes of the problem) in the knowledge database stored in the computer. The physician is given invaluable guidance from a thorough review of the possibilities.

Diagnostic couplers, as well as baseline and management couplers, are annotated with comments which provide the published background, competing theories, and the rationale for alternatives presented.

management problem knowledge coupler   A class of PKCouplers used when the cause of the patient's complaint is known and the problem becomes one of treatment. The management PKCoupler gives guidance as to alternative treatment paths. It takes into account any other problems the patient may have, and other treatments which may complicate the picture, giving the pros and cons of the alternatives, such as contraindications, relative probability of success, side-effects, and cost. Management PKCouplers use the same technique of collecting information from the patient (a structured questionnaire) and coupling it with the relevant literature as do the diagnosis and baseline couplers.

triage problem knowledge coupler   A newer class of PKCouplers which uses the same principles as the others. However, a triage coupler is used at the door to route a patient, as quickly as possible, to the most appropriate care. With a triage coupler, the physician's triage assistant first elicits information about the patient's reasons (problems) for seeking health or medical care, including the problem's onset, history, severity, and other relevant factors. Instead of the literature as the source of knowledge against which to couple the patient's profile, hosever, a triage coupler must be custom-tailored to the situation where it is to be employed. Its knowledge base for an office practice, for example, includes such information as the physician's kind of practice, the office's resources (such as laboratory and x-ray, and allied health professionals available), office hours, alternate physicians, and so on. Decision options might be, for example, direct hospitalization, referral to the emergency department, an office appointment immediately, an office appointment after indicated laboratory, X-ray, or other procedures, or an elective office visit.

Plans are under way to expand this triage concept to one-stop shopping for health care for an entire community.

problem-oriented medical record (POMR) See *problem-oriented medical record (POMR)* under *medical record*.

proceduralist A physician in whose specialty the performance of procedures, diagnostic or therapeutic, such as endoscopies and surgical operations, are a significant element. Physicians who are not proceduralists have no specific label, but their services are often described as "cognitive". Despite advent of the resource-based relative value scale (RBRVS) system in physician payment reform (PPR), the medical community still feels that the services provided by proceduralists are rewarded more highly than are cognitive services.

procedure In medicine, something which is "done" or "carried out" for a patient by a physician or other person. A procedure is usually discrete, and a relatively short time is required for its execution. Procedures are generally either diagnostic or therapeutic (treatment). A diagnostic procedure would be the taking of an X-ray or blood pressure, while a therapeutic procedure might be anything from removing a splinter from a finger to an extensive operation such as repair of a hernia.   A given operation, which might be called a "procedure," is often actually several procedures, and the array of procedures which make up a given operation will vary from patient to patient. For example, cholecystectomy (gall bladder removal) for one patient may include "exploration of the common bile duct," while for another patient, this procedure may be omitted. For this reason, a proper description of an operation requires that its procedures be listed.   For the purposes of health care financing (charges and payments for procedures), a hernia repair "procedure" might also include both preoperative and postoperative care. For more information about procedures in financing terminology, see *service*.

operating room procedure A term which, on its face, describes a surgical treatment of a patient, performed in the hospital's operating room. However, the term has a special function under the prospective payment system (PPS): if a patient has an "operating room procedure," that patient is placed in a different payment category than a patient in the same Major Diagnostic Category (MDC) who does not have an operating room procedure. For the purpose of making this allocation of patients, an arbitrary list of procedures (actually, a list of procedure codes) has been established by the Health Care Financing Administration (HCFA). If the patient's data set submitted for payment has a code shown on the HCFA's list as an operating room procedure, that patient is considered to have had an operating room procedure, no matter where the procedure was actually done.

procedure capture The mechanisms by which one given health care facility (a hospital, laboratory, or imaging service, for example) or specialist physician is selected in preference to another. Since such "procedure services" are the results of referral, primarily from physicians, "procedure capture" really is the sum of the efforts to persuade the referring person to make the referral to the institution or specialist seeking more business.

process The things done (for a patient, for example). It is commonly stated in quality management that three things can be measured: structure (resources or organization), process, and outcome. "Structure" refers to resources and organization. "Outcome" is a somewhat vague term that presumably refers to the results of the process. There is a tendency on the part of some individuals to take an "either-or" position, to the effect that one need only be concerned with one of the three dimensions. This tendency is not logical; all three must be considered. Clearly, certain structure is needed; and equally clearly, there is no way to change outcome except through changing process, since "outcome 'tells on' process."

product Something which is made (or grown). Often used in a marketing context to refer to whatever is sold to the consumer; in this context, "product" may mean either a tangible item or a service.

product liability See *product liability* under *liability*.

product line A term now being used in health care to denote the kinds of services offered by a health care institution, including, for example, the kinds of patients (defined by their diagnoses, procedures required, and age limitations accepted for care). For example, a hospital's product line might include three "products"—acute care, hospice care, and home health care—and might specifically exclude another product, obstetric care.

productivity The relationship between the number of units of service provided or products produced per unit of labor (or other cost) required, per unit of time. Productivity is said to increase in a hospital, for example, when patient stay can be reduced for a given illness with no sacrifice in quality and no increase in labor. On a larger scale, a hospital is sometimes considered more productive than another when it uses fewer employees, or has a lower cost per day.

products of ambulatory care (PAC) A classification developed by the New York State Ambulatory Care Reimbursement Demonstration Project in 1985 as a "sophisticated ambulatory care product definition." There are 24 PAC categories, into which patient visits are allocated by computer depending on "who the patient is" (type of problem presented) and what is done (resources received).

professional A worker whose occupation required them to complete a special educational or training program.

health care professional May mean an individual who is licensed, such as a physician, registered nurse (RN), or pharmacist, or it can refer to any worker in health care who has completed the required special training or education in their field. Whether or not a health professional needs to be licensed or certified depends on state law. For example, many "allied health professionals" may be well trained but not licensed. And, of course, some individuals may call themselves "professional" with little or no training. For example, there are no minimum requirements to be a "nutritionist," so anyone can call him or herself one. For some purposes—in a state or federal law, or in hospital policy, for instance—the word "professional" may be more precisely defined.

Professional Activity Study (PAS) The prototype hospital discharge abstract system. PAS is a program offered to hospitals by the Commission on Professional and Hospital Activities (CPHA). It uses abstracts of hospital medical records from enrolled hospitals as input to a database, and provides hospitals with indexes of their medical records and statistics on hospital performance. The database is also available for computer research on hospital activities, epidemiology, and health care studies. PAS offers case mix management information and other services to member hospitals.

professional association (PA)   See *professional corporation* under *corporation.*

professional service corporation (PSC)   See *professional corporation* under *corporation.*

Professional Standards Review Organization (PSRO)   An organization established under federal law to review medical necessity, appropriateness, and quality of services provided to beneficiaries of the Medicare, Medicaid, and maternal and child health (MCH) programs. These organizations were physician-sponsored. They have now been replaced in function by Peer Review Organizations (PROs) under the current federal program for the administration of Medicare.

profile   A statistical report showing certain predefined information about a given subject. The most common profiles in health care are physician profiles, which display such information as the numbers of patients cared for, their average length of stay in the hospital, the physician's use of various drugs and other treatments, and, more recently, the physician's *expensiveness*. Physicians are compared with each other on these attributes in an effort to encourage efficiency and frugality. See also *report card.*

profit   Excess of income over expense. Actually means an increase in assets. The word "gain" is often used in nonprofit corporations as a substitute for the word "profit."

prognosis   The physician's forecast as to the patient's future course. The prognosis is based on the usual course of progression of or recovery from a given disease or injury, modified by the physician's estimation of the patient's condition and other factors and their effects. A patient will have several prognoses covering length of illness, survival, recovery of function, and so on.

program evaluation and review technique (PERT)   A process to identify the accomplishments of programs and the time and resources required to move from one accomplishment to the next. The PERT diagram shows the sequence and interrelationship of activities from the beginning to the end of a project. See *critical path.*

Program of All-Inclusive Care for the Elderly (PACE)   A program, begun by the federal government in 1986, in which comprehensive long-term care programs are being conducted and studied as to their cost effectiveness. Initial reports are that such programs reduce the acute care hospital care required for their participants.

program-related investment (PRI)   A short-term (from one to ten year) loan from a foundation or other philanthropic organization to a nonprofit organization which is eligible for grants or charitable contributions. Nonprofit organizations often have difficulty in obtaining loans through normal channels because such organizations typically do not show profit margins, which the usual lending institutions see as essential in eligible borrowers. Recipients of PRIs may use the PRIs as collateral for obtaining loans through banks, as flexible lines of credit, or for other purposes. PRIs are only available for purposes which fall within the lending foundation's granting policy.

progressive patient care   A system of organizing patient care in the hospital in which the hospital establishes patient care units ready to provide different intensities of care (for example, intensive, intermediate, and self-care), and moves patients from unit to unit as they progress in their illnesses.

projection   In statistics, a calculated estimate for a whole calculated from data for a part of the whole, or an estimate of a future situation based on information currently available. The term "projection" is often used when sampling has given information from a part of a whole (for example, a population), and a projection is made as to the actual situation in the whole population. For example, a candidate's actual performance in opinion polls is "projected" from the response of a sample of voters.

proportion   A specific type of ratio in which the numerator is a part of the denominator. Proportions are always between 0 and 1 (inclusive). They are often expressed as rates such as percentages.

proprietary   For-profit and privately owned and managed.

prospective   Pertaining to the future. When used to refer to prospectively collected data in a research study, "prospective" means that special care is taken that the desired data are obtained from all individuals starting as of a given date.

prospective payment   A term often used as a misnomer for prospective pricing. "Prospective pricing" is the term which more accurately denotes the intent of the payment system currently being used for Medicare, which is discussed under *prospective payment system (PPS)*.

Under some circumstances, prospective payment for goods or services is made in advance (prepayment), either in whole or in partial payments, with adjustments made to the total when the actual amount due is determined. Payment in advance provides cash flow for the payee.

Prospective Payment Assessment Commission (ProPaC)   An advisory body established under Medicare to give advice and assistance to the Health Care Financing Administration (HCFA) on matters pertaining to the prospective payment system (PPS) under which Medicare operates. Advice from ProPaC is not binding on HCFA.

prospective payment system (PPS)   The name given the system currently in use for paying for services for Medicare patients (payment for patients "by Diagnosis Related Groups (DRGs)"). The idea is that patients are classified into categories (in this case, DRGs) for which prices are negotiated or imposed on the hospital in advance; thus it is actually "prospective pricing" rather than "prospective payment." At present PPS is only applied to hospital care, not physician care, although the idea is the same as a single fixed "package fee" which includes prenatal care, delivery, and postpartum care for a maternity patient, or the inclusion of preoperative care, operation, and postoperative care for an appendectomy patient within one fixed physician's fee. (In fact, the package fee concept is inherent in Physicians' Current Procedural Terminology (CPT), published by the American Medical Association (AMA)). PPS, while not mandated by federal law for payers other than Medicare, is being applied to patients under other health care plans.

PPS is sometimes referred to as the "DRG system." (The letters "PPS" are sometimes translated, incorrectly, to mean a prospective reimbursement system.)

prospective pricing Setting (or agreeing upon) prices in advance for the furnishing of a product or service. This is in direct contrast with the concept of reimbursement, in which the service or product is provided first, and then the provider is paid whatever it cost. The prospective payment system (PPS) adopted for Medicare, and applied also for other payers, is the most widespread example of prospective pricing.

The first step in prospective pricing is the definition of the product or service for which the price is to be set. Thus the Diagnosis Related Group (DRG) system of classification of patients, used in the PPS, is the first step in that prospective pricing application. The definition of procedures in Physicians' Current Procedural Terminology (CPT) could be a first step toward prospective pricing for physician services. Prospective pricing facilitates budgeting on the part of payers, since only the units of service or product likely to be needed have to be estimated or predicted; the cost of each unit is fixed in advance. On the other hand, prospective pricing increases the budgeting problems of the provider, since the provider is now at risk and must plan much more carefully or else lose on the prospectively priced "transaction" (of course, the provider may also gain on the transaction).

prospective pricing system (PPS) A sometimes translation of "PPS," which is generally translated to mean "prospective payment system." "Prospective pricing system" is, however, a more appropriate description of this payment system. See *prospective pricing*.

prospective reimbursement See *prospective reimbursement* under *reimbursement*.

protocol A plan of treatment or management. As used currently in hospital finance and quality management, a "protocol" typically means that, for a patient with a given problem, certain diagnostic and treatment procedures and length of stay are expected.

reverse protocol A term coined for the proposition that a given diagnostic or therapeutic procedure implies that a certain kind of diagnosis or problem must have been presented by the patient. For example, administration of a certain drug should have been explained by a class of disease (or prophylaxis) for which the drug was an appropriate treatment. Failure to find such a disease in the record would indicate an error in documentation or inappropriate use of the drug.

provider A hospital or other health care institution or health care professional which provides health care services to patients. A "provider" may be a single hospital, an individual, a group or organization, or even the government.

The Institute of Medicine (IOM) recommends restricting the use of the term "provider" to a system of healthcare, and using the term "clinician" for the individual health professional.

provider-driven system See *provider-driven system* under *economic system*.

Provider Reimbursement Review Board (PRRB)   A panel of five members appointed by the Secretary of the Department of Health and Human Services (DHHS), to which a provider may appeal a decision of a fiscal intermediary denying payment for services under Medicare.

provider service network (PSN)   A health care organization proposed in the (fall 1995) Republican House Medicare reform proposal. A PSN is operated by providers and is funded in part by the capital contributions of its members. It requires all members to provide health care to Medicare beneficiaries, and it receives the compensation on behalf of the members and distributes it among them. A PSN is given some antitrust protection under the bill with regard to establishment of fee schedules and the conduct of the network. A PSN is designed to operate like an HMO, offering HMO services and assuming risk, but is to be exempt from being regulated as an insurance company.

provider-sponsored organization (PSO)   A type of provider service network (PSN) proposed in the House of Representatives Republican Medicare reform proposal (Fall 1995). A PSO could be established and enter into business without the necessity of obtaining state licensure as an insurance (such licensure is required for other types of health care plans). The state could issue a certificate that the PSO meets federal requirements. The PSO would not be subject to any state law imposing capitalization or insolvency requirements that prevent it from doing business.

proxy   Someone who stands in for another person and is authorized to act on that person's behalf. See *health care proxy* under *advance directive*.

PSN   See *provider service network*.

psychographics   The analysis of populations on the basis of certain characteristics of individuals, specifically their attitudes, values, and lifestyles. The psychographic attributes of individuals are obtained by surveys or forms of psychometric testing. Such analyses are extensions of demographics. The attributes involved are not what are usually considered demographic; the analyses combine the psychographic data with demographic data. For example, it may be essential for some purposes to know the social consciousness (a psychographic item) of a population as it relates to various age and sex groups (demographic items).

Public Citizen Health Research Group (PCHRG)   An independent membership organization founded in 1971 by Sidney Wolfe, MD, and Ralph Nader (who was associated with PCHRG until 1982). PCHRG publishes a monthly newsletter, *Health Letter*, and states that its purpose is "to empower patients and to improve the safety and health of the workplace."

public health   The organized efforts on the part of society to reduce disease and premature death, and the disability and discomfort produced by disease and other factors, such as injury or environmental hazards. Public health is also a branch of preventive medicine, a medical specialty. Specialization in public health also occurs in engineering, nursing, nutrition, law, and other disciplines.

Public Health Service (PHS)   The organization within the Department of Health and Human Services (DHHS) which promotes physical and mental health, establishes national health policy, works with other countries regarding global health problems, conducts research, and so forth. Its components are perhaps better known. They include, among others:

> Agency for Toxic Substances and Disease Registry
> Alcohol, Drug Abuse, and Mental Health Administration
> Centers for Disease Control and Prevention (CDC)
> Food and Drug Administration (FDA)
> Health Resources and Services Administration (HRSA)
> Indian Health Service (IHS)
> National Institutes of Health (NIH)
> Office of the Surgeon General of the United States

public relations   The efforts to communicate with the hospital's audiences and constituencies and to enhance the hospital's image.

Q

quality-adjusted life-year (QALY)   A measure proposed to be used in economic analyses of the benefits of various procedures and programs.

quality and resource management (QRM)   A term being used in some hospitals to indicate that quality management and the conservation of resources are seen as a single topic, or at least, topics which are closely interrelated. Such hospitals may have, for example, quality management, utilization review, risk management, and infection control under the "QRM department" headed by the "QRM Director."

quality assurance (QA)   The efforts to determine the quality of care (find out the quality being provided), to develop and maintain programs to keep it an at acceptable level (quality control), and to institute improvements when the opportunity arises or the care does not meet the desired standard of care (medical) (quality improvement).

The term "quality assurance" is being replaced by "quality management." The advantages of the term "quality management" are: (1) there is no implication of a "guarantee," an idea which may be suggested by the use of the word "assurance," which is sometimes used as a synonym for "insurance"; and (2) "quality management" is more accurate, since the achievement of quality depends on people carrying out their responsibilities without error, and getting people to perform is the task of management.

Quality Assurance Monitor (QAM)   A part of the Professional Activity Study (PAS) of the Commission on Professional and Hospital Activities (CPHA). The care of patients, as reflected in their computerized discharge abstracts, is compared with standards established by clinical specialty societies, and the findings are displayed for use in hospital quality management.

quality circle   A group, formerly called a "quality control circle," which deals with concerns that relate to the quality of performance or quality of work life. There are six "non-negotiable" characteristics of a group which must be present if it is to be called a quality circle: (1) the group must be small; and (2) composed of individuals in the same work area (of a hospital, for example); (3) it must be voluntary; (4) it must consider problems (or opportunities for improvement) which the group itself selects; (5) the problems must affect the quality of work life or the quality of performance; and (6) the circle must propose solutions to management.

A quality circle is not to be confused with a committee or task force, both of which are appointed (not voluntary) and work on assigned tasks rather than self-selected tasks. Morale, productivity, and quality of performance are typically improved by the activities of quality circles. The groups often carry locally determined titles rather than being named "quality circles." Synonym(s): quality control circle.

quality control (QC)   The sum of all the activities which prevent unwanted change in quality. In the health care setting, quality control requires a repeated series of feedback loops which monitor and evaluate the care of the individual patient (and other systems in the health care process). These feedback loops involve checking the care being delivered against standards of care, the identification of any problems or opportunities for improvement, and prompt corrective action, so that the quality is maintained.

quality function   The sum of all the activities, wherever performed, through which the hospital achieves the quality of care it provides. This usage is comparable to speaking of the "fiscal function," which is the sum of the activities, wherever performed, through which the hospital achieves fiscal soundness. The term "quality function" is replacing "quality assurance function."

quality improvement (QI)   The sum of all the activities which create desired change in quality. In the health care setting, quality improvement requires a feedback loop which involves the identification of patterns of the care of patients (or of the performance of other systems involved in care), the analysis of those patterns in order to identify opportunities for improvement (or instances of departure from standards of care, and then action to improve the quality of care for future patients. An effective quality improvement system results in stepwise increases in quality of care. Quality control, with which quality improvement is sometimes confused, is the sum of all the activities which prevent unwanted change in quality.

continuous quality improvement (CQI)   As used in health care today, CQI means the application of industrial quality management theory in the health care setting, based upon principles of quality "gurus" W. Edwards Deming and Joseph M. Juran. While traditional "quality control" theories seek out "fault" and attempt improvement by exhorting people to change their behavior, continuous improvement seeks to understand processes and revise them on the basis of data about the processes themselves. CQI sees "problems" as opportunities for improvement. The CQI process involves a project-by-project approach to systematically improve quality, not just to maintain the status quo. A major project in this area is the National Demonstration Project on Quality Improvement in Health Care, sponsored by a grant from the John A. Hartford Foundation, being conducted by Harvard Community Health Plan in Brookline, Massachusetts, in conjunction with the Juran Institute (a quality consulting and education firm in Wilton, Connecticut).

quality improvement project (QIP)   One activity in the process of continuous quality improvement (CQI). Each project involves a process which has been identified as deserving improvement, and which has been given priority (prioritizing of effort is critical in CQI). For each project, a team is assigned consisting of representatives from all departments involved in the process targeted for improvement, along with support from senior management. The team studies the process, comes up with theories for improvement, tests the theories, puts successful theories into place, and also puts into place measures to assure that the improved quality is maintained.

Examples of hospital QIPs conducted as part of the National Demonstration Project on Quality Improvement in Health Care are reduction in medication errors; reduction of unbilled drugs (thereby increasing revenues); reduction of delays in surgery starting times (with a corresponding savings in hospital staff overtime expenses).

quality management (QM)   Efforts to determine the quality of care, to develop and maintain programs to keep it at an acceptable level (quality control), to institute improvements when the opportunity arises or the care does not meet standards (quality improvement), and to provide, to all concerned, the evidence required to establish confidence that quality is being managed and maintained at the desired level. (These are the same elements that are inherent in industrial quality management.) The advantages of the term "quality management" over "quality assurance" are: (1) there is no implication of a "guarantee," an idea which may be suggested by the use of the word "assurance," which is sometimes used as a synonym for "insurance"; and (2) "quality management" is more accurate, since the achievement of quality depends on people carrying out their responsibilities without error, and getting people to perform is the task of management.

total quality management (TQM)   Used to describe a philosophy (and actions) of an organization which is dedicated to continuous quality improvement (CQI) throughout the organization. A hospital with total quality management will, for example, set specific quality goals, choose a number of high priority quality improvement projects (QIPs), make quality improvement part of job descriptions throughout the organization and legitimize time spent on quality improvement, provide necessary resources (financial and otherwise), provide essential training for staff involved, and formally recognize quality improvement efforts. Total quality management requires commitment and personal involvement of senior management. It should be emphasized that quality control (prevention of unwanted change in quality) must be maintained in parallel with quality improvement, and that quality control demands the same energy commitment as does quality improvement.

quality management audit   See *quality management audit* under *audit*.

quality of care   The degree of conformity with accepted principles and practices (standards), the degree of fitness for the patient's needs, and the degree of attainment of achievable outcomes (results), consonant with the appropriate allocation or use of resources. The phrase "quality of care" carries the concept that quality is not equivalent to "more" or "higher technology" or higher cost. The "degree of conformity" with standards focuses on the provider's performance, while the "degree of fitness" for the patient's needs indicates that the patient may present conditions which override strict conformity with otherwise prescribed procedures.

quality of life (QOL)   A condition often given as one attribute or dimension of health. It is ill-defined, depending on the individual and his goals, the social setting and expectations (often of others), and other factors. The goal of much of health care is stated to be improved quality of life. One of the most challenging problems in health care is to measure quality of life so that (1) improvement can be identified, and (2) it can be used as a factor in cost-benefit analysis. There is a real danger that inability to express quality of life in numerical terms will mean that much valuable care will not be available because quality of life cannot be given a value and therefore cannot be used to justify the expenditure (to end up with a positive cost-benefit ratio (see *ratio*) rather than a negative ratio); consequently, mere survival could be the measure.

An illustration is the debate over the "value" of some coronary bypass operations; patients in some studies have not shown significantly greater life expectancies with the operation than without it, but the patients operated on regularly testify to their pleasure with their relief from pain. In some instances (intractable pain or helplessness, for example), life itself is of such low quality to the individual that he may prefer not to live.

health-related quality of life (HRQOL)   A number of aspects of quality of life (QOL) which are related to health, such as mental health, perceived physical health, and social and role functioning. The relevant aspects are sometimes developed under the headings of "physical well-being, perceived health, emotional well-being, home management, work functioning, recreation, social functioning, and sexual functioning."

quality of life scale   A method designed to measure the quality of life of an individual, based upon one or more aspects of life and health. More than 50 such measurement methods have been developed. Some investigators have developed weighting methods by which to consolidate the data from a number of scale measurements into a single score for an individual.Some of these scales, both single-characteristic and consolidated, are described below:

quality staircase   A method of representing the results of quality improvement efforts. Joseph M. Juran in the industrial setting has represented quality improvement as an ever-rising spiral, an inclined plane. The processes involved in making the product or providing the service are constantly monitored and, as opportunities for improvement are identified, changes are made which result in breakthroughs to higher levels of quality. In certain respects, the concept of a staircase is more appropriate than that of a spiral, since breakthroughs actually improve quality in steps rather than in a continuous fashion.

quill pen law   A law which requires records to be maintained in written, rather than electronic, form.

R

rate (charge)   A financial term referring to a hospital or other institution's charges. Typically rates are "fixed" in that they are for specified services, and the same rate is charged to all individuals or to purchasers of a given class (such as Medicare patients). For example, a hotel could have different rates for senior citizens, commercial travellers, and the general public.

blended rate   A term used in the prospective payment system (PPS) of Medicare to designate a rate which is formed by combining the hospital-specific rate and the federal Medicare rate.

hospital-specific rate   A term used in the Medicare prospective payment system (PPS) in the computation of the hospital's payment. This rate is "blended" with the federal Medicare rate in certain circumstances.

inclusive rate   A prospectively established rate for a day of care which includes all hospital services that may be required, regardless of their nature or cost.

interim rate   A temporary rate used in a reimbursement system which periodically makes payments to the hospital on the basis of an estimated figure. The rate is subsequently adjusted retrospectively to reflect actual expenses: additional payments are made to the hospital, or the hospital refunds part of the payment it received; and corrections are made to future rates as appropriate. Using an interim rate provides operating cash for the hospital in a "retrospective reimbursement" payment system, where payment is based on actual costs as determined at the end of the fiscal period.

per diem rate   A rate established by dividing total costs (plus a percentage for excess of income over expenses) by the total number of inpatient days of care for the same period. Thus the per diem rate is the same for each patient, regardless of the patient's illness, its severity, or the diagnostic or therapeutic measures required.

room rate   Same as "daily service charge": the dollar amount the hospital charges for one day of inpatient care for "room and board" and basic nursing and hospital care. The term is not used when, for example, an inclusive rate system is employed since, in that case, the daily rate includes more than these items.

rural rate   A type of rate computed by Medicare for hospitals Medicare classifies as rural.

urban rate   A type of rate computed by Medicare for hospitals Medicare classifies as urban.

rate (ratio)   A ratio or proportion, often expressed as a percentage (per 100), but which may also be expressed per 1,000, per 10,000, per 100,000, or even per million. These "per" numbers are called the "base." Thus a rate expressed per 100,000 is said to have 100,000 as the base. The base chosen is usually large enough to insure that the rate will be expressed in whole numbers; the more rare the event, the larger the base chosen. A death rate of 7 per 10,000 is easier to understand than a rate of 0.07 percent (although both actually give the same information).

rating   The determination, by an actuary, of the health care risk (actuarial) for a given group in order to establish the insurance premium to be charged.

community rating   Establishment of insurance or health care plan premiums on the basis of the average health care demands of an entire community (or enrolled population), so that all individuals in the community pay the same premium. A person's sex, age, or physical condition is not allowed to raise the premium, so there is no financial penalty for having a history of illness. Many states require HMOs to use community rating in setting their premiums. The alternative is experience rating.

adjusted community rating (ACR)   A way of setting group rates for the next year based on the actual experience of a group (enrolled population) during the past year. The average use of services for all members is used to predict the future use by the group. This adjustment factor is applied to the basic community rates, yielding the adjusted community rates. This method is used by many managed care plans to set premiums at a level predicted to be sufficient to cover the costs of the group's use of services the following year. However, after the rate is set, it may not be changed nor adjusted retroactively.

experience rating   Establishment of insurance or health care plan premiums on the basis of an actuarial analysis of the sex and age composition of the group, type of industry, and other factors, which are used to set the initial premiums., calls for lower premiums for healthier subsets of the population and higher for subsets, such as the elderly, who require more care In subsequent years, the actual record of the group may be used to modify the rating and the premiums. Often preexisting conditions are taken into the analysis and may be cause for rejection of enrollment of certain individuals. Actuarial analyses would, for example, give weights to sex and age: A preponderance of young males would point to a lower rate than females because of the lower obstetric exposure, but this would be countered by the higher accidental injury rates for males. Actuarial analysis is a complicated science. Experience rating is, of course, sought by employers of young, healthy individuals. The result is that the remainder of a given population, with poorer experience, pays more.

ratio   A value obtained by dividing one number (the numerator) by another (the denominator). See also *proportion*.

cost-benefit ratio   A mathematical expression of the benefits of a given service or the use of certain equipment compared with its costs. To develop such a ratio, both costs and benefits must be expressed in dollars, a task much easier for costs than benefits in many health care situations (improved quality of life may truly be a benefit, but expressing it in dollars is, at best, difficult). A ratio of 1.0 means that the benefits and costs are equal; a ratio over 1.0 means that the benefits exceed the costs; and a ratio under 1.0 means that the costs exceed the benefits.

cost-to-charge ratio A term used in finance, which shows whether a charge for a given product or service is set so that it covers the cost. A ratio of 1.0 means that the cost and charge are identical; a ratio greater than 1.0 means that the charge does not recover the cost; and a ratio less than 1.0 means that the charge exceeds the cost. See also *ratio of costs to charges*.

ratio of costs to charges (RCC) A method of estimating costs in accounting. There is generally a desire that charges for health care reflect the costs of that care. This is fairly easy to achieve globally, that is, the total costs for a hospital, say, for a year can be ascertained and the charges or reimbursement can be matched to those costs. It is also easy to learn the total costs and the total charges for a revenue producing department, such as radiology. Typically, the total charges exceed the total costs, and the ratio between these two figures is easily obtained.

Since it may be virtually impossible (or far more costly than can be justified) to find the actual costs of specific procedures and services, such as the cost of a chest X-ray, an approximation is made. Under the RCC approach, this is done by simply multiplying the charge for the procedure by the cost/charge ratio for the department, and using the resulting dollar amount as (an estimate of) the cost of the procedure. For example, if the (total) costs for the department are $100,000 and the (total) charges are $200,000, the ratio, $100,000/$200,000, is 0.5. Applying the RCC method, then, all charges would be multiplied by this ratio, and a chest X-ray, say, for which there is a $50.00 charge would be considered to have a $25.00 cost.

rationing A process of withholding goods or services when they are in short supply. Rationing of health care is, of course, in one sense in effect, since it is not possible to provide all the care which has been proven effective to all the individuals who might benefit from it. In the climate of health care reform, discussion revolves around the problems of deciding the basis on which the limited financial and other resources will be allocated; on who will get what care there is. One method of rationing is financial: when the money runs out the care stops. This is first-come first-served. Another rationing method is to identify certain groups of patients, such as Medicare and Medicaid, as eligible for the benefits. Other methods have been proposed, such as cutting benefits off on the basis of age. Perhaps the most scientific and fair method proposed is the "Oregon plan" in which there is an *explicit* list of patient-care "problem-treatment (diagnosis-treatment) pairs," ranked as to their benefits to the individuals and to society. Those most beneficial, ranked highest, are funded first, and actuarial methods determine how far down the list the available funds will go. A line is drawn at that point, and lower ranked services are not paid for from the given fund source. See *Oregon plan*.

RBRVS Resource-based relative value scale (RBRVS), see under *relative value scale*.

reappointment The process of formally continuing the medical staff membership of a physician or other health care professional, along with specific privileges. After the initial appointment to the staff, reappointment must take place at regular intervals (usually every year or two). During the reappointment process, the performance of the professional is evaluated, so that a proper determination can be made regarding renewal (or increase or decrease) of clinical privileges. If privileges are to be decreased or discontinued, certain due process procedures are required.

record   See *database* and *medical record*.

recovery (get well)   Regaining of the condition of health or function which preceded the occurrence of a disease or disability. Used in the context of postoperative care, recovery refers to the period of time immediately following surgery, during which the patient is closely monitored in the recovery room until stabilized. Patients stay in the recovery room until they are ready to be returned to their hospital room (if inpatients) or to go home (if outpatients).

recovery (get money)   The money awarded by a court to the successful plaintiff in a lawsuit. The term can also mean the amount of money actually collected.

recredentialing   Determining and certifying as to the competency of a physician or other professional at some time after the initial determination of his or her qualification for licensure or hospital privileges. Recredentialing is required at periodic intervals in some hospitals and health care organizations. It is also under consideration by several states as a procedure to be followed at the time of renewal of licenses (most states simply require payment of a fee). As being discussed with regard to renewal of license, "recredentialing" does not rely on evidence of meeting continuing education requirements or written examination as to knowledge. The focus is on the physician's actual performance. Under consideration are computer-based "clinical" testing and the use of hospital quality review records. In the case of physicians whose practice is entirely in their offices, an office audit system (now used in Canada) is under consideration. See also *credentialing*.

recuse   To reject or challenge an individual's qualification to serve in a given capacity, usually on the basis of conflict of interest or known bias. Usually used with respect to a judge or juror. Individuals may also recuse themselves voluntarily, to avoid the appearance of impropriety.

Redefining Progress   A nonprofit public-policy organization in San Francisco, one of whose goals is to develop a new measure of the economic condition of the nation; see *Genuine Progress Indicator (GPI)).*

referral   The sending of a patient by one physician (the referring physician) to another physician (or some other resource) either for consultation or for care. Specialist care (secondary care) is ordinarily on referral from a primary care physician or another specialist. Care of the patient is given back to the referring physician if the referral was for consultation or where the specialist has completed the care required; otherwise the patient is transferred to the specialist, who takes over responsibility for the patient.   For example, if a primary care physician refers a patient suspected of having appendicitis to a surgeon (and the surgeon also diagnoses appendicitis), the surgeon customarily performs the appendectomy and returns the patient to the referring physician afterward. However, if a general internist refers a problem diabetic patient to an endocrinologist (specialist in diabetes and other endocrine diseases), the referral might result in the permanent transfer of the patient.

referral center   A rural hospital classified as such by the federal government, for purposes of reimbursement under the Medicare prospective payment system (PPS).

regional alliance, regional health alliance   See *regional alliance, regional health alliance* under *health alliance (HA)*.

registry (data)   A central agency where data from an institution or specific geographic area can be collected and made available for study and, in the health care field, sometimes made available for assisting in patient care management. An illustration of the latter use is in sending reminders to patients when follow-up examinations are scheduled (for example, in the case of tumors).

regression   A statistical method used to measure and express the effect one variable, the "independent variable," has on another variable, the "dependent variable." A physician may want to increase the concentration of a drug in a patient's blood. The question: if the physician doubles the dose of a given drug (the dosage of the drug is the independent variable, because it can be controlled), will it double the concentration of the drug (the dependent variable) in the patient's blood, or will it less than double, and will the effects vary from patient to patient? Regression is used to help answer this question. A collection of data on drug dosages (related to patients' weights, for example) and the same patients' blood concentrations of the drug are analyzed by an appropriate regression method. The analysis will tell the relationship between doses and blood levels—not only the probable increases (or decreases, which could happen) in proportion to dosage, but also the ranges of response which are likely to occur.

A common form of regression is a "linear regression," in which the "model" chosen for the analysis is a linear equation.

regulation   A rule or procedure made by a governmental agency, and having the force of law, as contrasted with an administrative guideline , which is merely advisory.

Another type of regulation is that adopted by a corporation or association as part of its internal rules and regulations. However, this latter type of regulation is seldom spoken of separate from the phrase, "rules and regulations" of the corporation.

rehabilitation   Efforts to assist the patient to achieve and maintain her optimal level of function, self-care, and independence, after or in correction of a disability. The disability may be physical, mental, or emotional.

rehabilitation potential   Realistic goals for the individual patient with respect to (1) management of the patient's specific health problems and (2) achievement of self-care, independence, and emotional well-being. These goals are set and stated by the attending physician for each patient at the time of admission to a rehabilitation hospital or long-term care facility (LTCF).

reimbursement   The payment to a hospital or other provider, after the fact, of an amount equal to the provider's expenses in providing a given service or product. The current trend is away from such a "blank check" approach and toward prospective pricing, that is, toward agreement in advance as to the amount which will be paid for the service or product in question. Several varieties of reimbursement are discussed in health care:

cost-based reimbursement Payment of all allowable costs incurred in the provision of care. The term "allowable" refers to the terms of the contract under which care is furnished.

prospective reimbursement A term sometimes used, incorrectly, instead of prospective pricing or prospective payment. See *prospective payment system (PPS)*. Also, "prospective reimbursement" is sometimes used to describe the prospectively estimated amount to be paid a hospital on a current schedule so that it will have operating cash, with the understanding that adjustments will be made later in the light of actual operating cost data. The concept is similar to that of the periodic interim payment (PIP).

retroactive reimbursement Additional payment to a provider for costs not considered at the time of original reimbursement.

retrospective reimbursement Payment based on actual costs as determined at the end of the fiscal period.

third party reimbursement (TPR) Payment for health care services by a third party such as an insurance company.

reimbursement specialist A person who is involved with working out the terms and details of reimbursement systems with third-party payers. Sometimes just refers to a person who prepares the statements and other materials needed to obtain reimbursement from third-party payers and insurers for services, and who maintains the related records. (Sometimes called insurance clerk).

reinsurance A type of insurance that insurance companies themselves buy for their own protection. Reinsurance further shares the risk. Health care insurances frequently reinsure themselves for specified, rare, and high priced risks, such as heart transplantation.

relative value scale (RVS) A numerical system (scale) designed to permit comparisons of the resources needed (or appropriate prices) for various units of service. The RVS is the compiled table of the relative value units (RVUs) for all the objects in the class for which it is developed.
  An RVS takes into account labor, skill, supplies, equipment, space, and other costs into an aggregate cost for each procedure or other unit of service. The aggregate cost is converted into the relative value unit (RVU) of the procedure or service by relating it to the cost of a procedure or service selected as the "base unit." For example, the developer of the RVS for laboratory work might decide to use the cost of a red blood count as the base unit. Its actual cost might be $5.00, but, as the base, its RVU would arbitrarily be set at 1.0. If a blood sugar estimation, then, actually cost $25.00, it would have an RVU value of 5.0 ($25.00 divided by $5.00) (the illustration is imaginary as to the prices given). If a urinalysis cost $3.00, it would have an RVU of 0.6.

resource-based relative value scale (RBRVS) A method of determining physicians' fees based on the time, training, skill, and other factors required to deliver various services. The term came into use in 1988 upon release of the report of a study commissioned by the Department of Health and Human Services (DHHS) and carried out under the direction of Harvard economist William Hsiao, PhD. See *relative value scale.*

relative value unit (RVU) The numerical value given to each procedure or other unit of service in a "relative value scale." See *relative value scale (RVS).*

reliability The degree of accuracy of results over a period of time, a number of trials, or among different observers or investigators. Also, the probability that a system will perform its function properly for a given period of time.

interrater reliability The degree of agreement among different persons (raters) expressing judgments (ratings) on the same data or observations.

intrarater reliability The degree of agreement among judgments (ratings) made by the same person (rater) on the same data or observations at different times.

remedy In law, something which a court (or a statute) grants to redress a wrong or make an injured person whole. The most common remedy is money. Another, less common remedy is an injunction (ordering the defendant to do something or stop doing something).

exclusive remedy A remedy provided by law which precludes a person from trying to obtain any kind of compensation other than that provided by the law. An example is workers' compensation, which is the exclusive remedy for on-the-job injuries; an injured worker who is entitled to receive workers' compensation benefits may not sue his employer for damages.

report card A generic term for performance statements pertaining to health care professionals and providers. Report cards are being issued increasingly by health care institutions, regulatory agencies, insurers, managed care organizations, accrediting bodies and others, giving information such as health care outcomes, costs, charges, severity of illness of patients, intensity of services, institution staffing, medical staff composition, patient satisfaction, provision of preventive services, and other data. Report cards may be designed for such purposes as internal information, for employers, or release to the public. The Joint Commission on the Accreditation of Healthcare Organizations (JCAHO) began releasing, on request, report cards giving details of its survey reports in December 1994.

required request law A law which requires hospitals to develop programs for asking families of deceased patients to donate the organs of the deceased for transplantation. Synonym(s): routine inquiry law.

Resource Utilization Groups (RUGs) II A case mix payment system used in New York state for long-term care patients under Medicare and Medicaid.

resource-based relative value scale (RBRVS) See *resource-based relative value scale (RBRVS)* under *relative value scale.*

respite care   Short term care (usually a few days) for a long-term care patient in order to provide a respite (rest and change) for those who have been caring for the patient, usually the patient's family. Respite care may involve hospitalization of the patient, or provision of round-the-clock care at home or in a nursing home as needed.

respondeat superior   "Let the master answer." A legal doctrine which makes an employer liable for the negligent acts of its employees, even though the employer was itself not negligent. Similarly, a principal is liable for the acts of its agent.

responsible party   The individual or organization responsible for placing a patient in a health care facility and ensuring that adequate care is given to that patient there. For example, a parent is usually the responsible party in the case of a child; the parent is not only responsible for the child receiving care, but also for the payment for that care. In less formal usage in the hospital, the term "responsible party" is used to mean simply "responsible for payment." Legally, there can be more than one "responsible party." For example, one person, such as a guardian, may be authorized to make treatment decisions, while another person may be responsible for payment.

rest home   A free-standing facility set up to provide care for patients who are unable to live independently, that is, who need assistance with the activities of daily living (ADL), and who may need occasional assistance from a professional nurse. Such professional nursing service is obtained from a visiting nurse. Regulations usually apply the designation of rest home to a facility with over, say, six beds, but as a practical matter it is usually not economical to operate a rest home with fewer than thirty or forty beds. A facility providing similar service to a smaller number of persons may be called (and licensed as) a "family care home" (FCH) or "adult foster home." Rest home was formerly called "custodial care home."

restructuring   Reorganization of a corporation (a hospital, for example) in order better to handle new functions and enterprises. The restructuring may involve the creation of several corporations where there was only one, consolidation or merger of corporations, establishment of foundations, and the like. Restructuring is often essential to achieve effective diversification.

retirement center   A facility which provides social activities to senior citizens, usually retired persons, who do not require health care. The provision of housing is not required for an institution or organization to be called a retirement center. A retirement center may furnish housing and may also have acute hospital and long-term care facilities, or it may arrange for acute and long-term care through affiliated institutions.

retroactive date   The date stipulated in a claims-made coverage policy as the earliest date an event may occur and be covered under that particular claims-made policy. For example, a policy for calendar year 1990 with a retroactive date of January 1, 1985, would cover an event occurring anytime on or after January 1, 1985, if the claim based on that event is made during 1990.

revenue   Increase in an organization's assets or a decrease in its liabilities during an accounting period. This is in contrast with income, which refers to money earned during an accounting period.

reverse protocol   See *reverse protocol* under *protocol*.

review   The processes of examination and evaluation.

admissions review   An evaluation of the appropriateness of the admission of the patient to the hospital. The admissions review determines whether the patient in question was in a condition which warranted use of the hospital, or could (or should) have been treated in some other setting (for example, at home or as an outpatient, or in a hospital more suited to managing his problem). Typically, the admissions review is carried out at or shortly after admission.

capital expenditure review (CER)   A process carried out by a state agency prior to granting permission to the hospital to incur a capital expenditure.

claims review   Retrospective review of hospital claims by a third party payer in order to determine the: (1) liability of the payer (whether the benefit was included in the contract); (2) eligibility of the beneficiary and the provider; (3) appropriateness of the service; and (4) appropriateness of the amount claimed.

concurrent review   Evaluation of medical necessity for admission and appropriateness of services, carried out while the patient is in the hospital (concurrent with the care). The advantage of concurrent review is that if any action (change in the care) is found to be necessary as a finding of the review, it can be taken while the patient is still in the hospital.

continued stay review   Concurrent review (review while the patient is in the hospital), conducted at a specified time after admission, for the purpose of determining the appropriateness of continuation of hospital care for the individual patient.

drug utilization review   Review of the use of drugs, either in the practice of a physician or in the hospital.

medical services review   Retrospective review of the use of services (and failure to use services), for both inpatients and outpatients, with respect to the medical appropriateness of the services and, in some situations, review of whether the services are included in the patient's insurance benefits.

peer review   See the separate listing of *peer review*.

preadmission review   Evaluation, prior to admission, of the necessity for elective hospitalization for the individual patient in question.

preprocedure review   A review of a case prior to the performance of a given procedure in order to determine (1) if the procedure is medically indicated, and (2) if the procedure could equally well be performed in an alternate setting.

rate review   Review by a regulatory agency of a hospital's budget and financial picture in order to determine the reasonableness of the hospital's proposed rates and rate changes. Rate review is also applied to rates for certain prepayment plans, such as Blue Cross/Blue Shield (BC/BS), depending on state laws.

utilization review (UR)   The examination and evaluation of the efficiency and appropriateness of any health care service. Often the term applies to a concurrent process, one carried out during hospitalization, for determination of the individual patient's need for continued stay.

right to die   The legal right to refuse life-saving or life-sustaining treatment. A competent adult has the legal right to refuse medical treatment, even if that treatment is essential to sustain life. Some refer to this right as the "right to die." The issue of the "right to die" arises in the situation where a person has a condition in which the quality of life is so intolerable that death, at least in the belief of that individual (or those responsible for that person), is preferable. If the person is conscious (and mentally competent), he or she may exercise the right to refuse treatment for him or herself; but if unconscious or otherwise incompetent, others must make the decision for him or her. Serious legal and ethical issues are involved in the latter case.

risk (financial)   A chance of monetary loss; direct exposure. A health care plan (for example, a health maintenance organization) is said to be at risk if it offers prepaid care for a given fee or premium. The plan is at risk because it must provide the care within the premium funds available, find the money elsewhere (the individual assets of the partners, for example), or suffer a loss.

risk (insurance)   Chance of loss, the type of which can usually be covered by insurance. To a health care institution, the risk may arise through general liability (such as a visitor slipping and falling on hospital premises) or professional liability (harm to a patient from medical or hospital care). It may also arise because of other hospital liability (antitrust violations, for example) or physical property damage.

risk (health)   The likelihood of disease, injury, or death among various groups of individuals and from different causes. Individuals are said to be "at risk" if they are in a group in which a given causal factor is present. Patients who smoke are at risk from smoking; patients undergoing appendectomy are at risk from this operation. This definition is that employed in public health.

risk (actuarial)   An actuary's statement of the risk presented by a group of individuals which is being considered for enrollment in health care insurance. This risk statement is the basis for rating the group, i.e., determining the insurance premium to be charged. For community rating, the risk statement is for the entire community; for experience rating, the statement is for a smaller group, such as the employees of a given corporation. See *rating*.

risk adjustment   The use of severity of illness measures to estimate the risk to which a patient is subject.

risk analysis   In connection with computer software, answering three questions: (1) what can go wrong; (2) how likely is it, and (3) what are the consequences of failure. There is a distinction between (1) a hazard, (2) a failure, (3) a risk, and (4) an accident.

risk contract   See *risk contract* under *contract*.

risk factors Factors in the individual's genetic and physical makeup, life-style and behavior, and environment which are known (or thought) to increase the likelihood of physical or mental problems. Risk factors are typically specific for given kinds of problems. For example, obesity, high blood pressure, high cholesterol, high blood sugar, and smoking are all considered risk factors for coronary artery disease (blood vessel disease in the heart), while several of these are also related to cerebrovascular disease (blood vessel disease in the brain). Risk factors for poisoning of children are such things as failure to properly store drugs and household chemicals. There are also risk factors which contribute to *getting* a risk factor: for example, people who live sedentary lives are more likely to have high blood pressure than those who are physically active.

risk management The process of minimizing risk insurance to an organization at a minimal cost in keeping with the organization's objectives. Risk management includes risk control and risk financing. Risk control involves: (1) developing systems to prevent accidents, injuries, and other adverse occurrences, and (2) attempting to handle events and incidents which do occur in such a manner that their cost is minimized. The latter might involve, for example, special attention to personal relations with the injured party, attempts to reach satisfactory settlement without lawsuit, and the like. Risk financing involves the procurement of adequate financial protection from loss, either through an outside insurance company or through some form of self-insurance.

risk pool A fund set up as a reserve for unexpected expenses in a prepaid health plan. Organizations which provide prepaid health care for a fixed fee typically set up such pools to cover, for example, unusually large demands for hospital care or specialist services.

high risk pool A fund set up to offer health insurance to small groups and individuals who have been denied coverage or whose medical history makes rates too high.

risk selection Action by a health care plan or insurer which seeks to enroll only healthy persons (low risk), thus reducing the risk to the plan. Of course, adverse selection results in enrollment of a group of persons who are below the norm in health, and thus likely to be more costly for the plan. Health care reform proposals would, along with requiring community rating, prevent risk selection.

risk sharing The division of financial risk among those furnishing the service. For example, if a hospital and group of physicians form a corporation to provide health care at a fixed price, they will ordinarily do it under an arrangement in which the hospital and physicians are both liable if the expenses exceed the revenue; that is, they share the risk.

Robert Wood Johnson Foundation Major philanthropic organization focusing on health care issues. RWJF addresses issues including access, delivery of care to the chronically ill, substance abuse, and escalating costs. See also *Alpha Center*, *Community Health Intervention Partnerships (CHIPs)* and *Partnership for Long Term Care (PLTC)*.

Robinson-Patman Act   A federal antitrust law which prohibits price discrimination. A seller cannot charge a buyer a discriminatory price and a buyer cannot knowingly benefit from such a price. The prohibition applies only to sales of goods. Discrimination may be justified in some cases if the seller can show a relationship between the discount and the cost of manufacture or delivery of the product (for example, in a volume discount), or if the discount is needed to meet the competition. The Robinson-Patman Act is an amendment to Section 2 of the Clayton Act. 15 U.S.C. secs. 13-13b.21(a) (1982).

An important exemption from the Robinson-Patman Act is that granted to non-profit hospitals (and certain other organizations) which purchase supplies for their own use. For example, "own use" has been interpreted to prohibit a hospital from selling prescription drugs (which it obtains at favorable prices) to the general public and outpatients coming in for refills, but to allow the hospital to sell or furnish drugs to inpatients, outpatients seen at the hospital, and physicians and employees and their families.

rooming-in   An organization of the maternity and newborn services of a hospital which permits the newborn to share the room with the mother.

RUGs   See *Resource Utilization Groups (RUGs) II.*

Rule of Reason   A doctrine in antitrust law which states that only unreasonable restraints of trade are prohibited. Thus, in most cases of alleged anticompetitive behavior, the specific facts must be examined to decide whether an antitrust violation has occurred. For example, an exclusive contract between a hospital and a group of radiologists is anticompetitive on its face; that is, it precludes other radiologists from practicing in the hospital. However, courts have decided, by applying the Rule of Reason, that such arrangements may be upheld for reasons of quality of care, administrative efficiency, or other valid institutional goals. By contrast, if the per se standard were applied, the exclusive contract would be illegal regardless of its purpose. In health care cases, courts have been more likely to apply the Rule of Reason analysis than they have been in other industries.

Rule of Rescue   The principle that saving a patient from imminent death has priority over any other medical duty. This "rule" is stated by some as a fact of the human psyche in connection with discussions of the rationing of health care.

rules and regulations   Official statements (statements authorized or commissioned by the governing body) as to the conduct of the organization's affairs in specific areas. In hospitals, the term often applies to statements which supplement the medical staff bylaws. Such rules and regulations have the force of the bylaws themselves, but contain more detail than would be appropriate in the bylaws; also, the process for their revision is less cumbersome than that for the revision of bylaws. For example, the bylaws could require the keeping of a medical record on each patient, while the rules and regulations could specify more detailed requirements concerning the content of medical records, promptness of completion, penalties for failure to comply, and so on.

RVS   See *relative value scale.*

RVU   See *relative value unit.*

Ryan White CARE (Comprehensive AIDS Resources Emergency Care) Act A 1990 federal act, named for an Indiana boy with AIDS, which was designed to help urban areas; now up for reauthorization when AIDS is also rural.

S

safe harbor regulations Regulations which describe certain acts or behaviors which will *not* be illegal under a specific law, even though they might overwise arguably be illegal. Federal safe harbor regulations specify certain joint ventures and other arrangements concerning hospitals and/or physicians which will not violate federal Medicare *fraud and abuse* laws.

safety-critical Systems whose failure can cause injury or death or damage to life-sustaining qualities of the earth. For example, a control system for radiation therapy dosage is a safety-critical system; its failure may result in radiation burns or death. A control system for a washing machine is likely to be mission-critical; its failure is likely to result merely in dirty clothes.

sample A part of a population, intended to be in some way representative of the population.

sampling A technique used in statistics in which a part of a whole is examined with the intent that the results of the examination can be taken as representing the condition of the whole. A large body of theory and experience has been developed as to various sampling methods (methods of drawing samples), and their reliability, that is, the trustworthiness of the projections made from them. In general, the more random the sample, the better (i.e., the more likely the sample will accurately reflect the condition of the whole). One example of sampling involves coal, which is sometimes sold on the basis of its heating value. Small quantities thought to represent the whole are analyzed, and payment is based on these analyses. The same principle is used in polls as to a political candidate's popularity: a sample of people are questioned and their responses are projected as representative of the whole population from which they were selected (for example, a city). Most skepticism about sampling revolves around whether the sample was a correct one for the purpose.

sanction A term used with two, opposite meanings: (1) a kind of permission or support; and (2) discipline, punishment, or prohibition. Only by the context can one determine which meaning is intended.

scoring A term used in connection with legislative budgeting in estimating the effects on revenue of tax policy changes, depending on their influence on behavior. *Static* scoring is used when no effect on behavior is expected from the change in tax policy; *dynamic* scoring is used when behavior is expected to change. Also called "cost estimating". An example of a behavioral change in response to tax policy has been the noticeable change to automobile leasing from purchasing as a response to the elimination of the deductibility of personal interest expense. The Congressional Budget Office (CBO) tends to use static scoring in its budget predictions.

screening (quality) A method for separating some kinds of things or patients from others. The term is often employed in one method of assessing quality of care, in which medical records of patients are subjected to a "screen" which isolates for detailed review the records of those with unusually long stays, or those with complications of care, for example.

generic screening Screening in which the criteria used to "screen" cases apply to patients regardless of their diagnoses and procedures employed; thus the criteria are "generic" rather than diagnosis- or procedure-specific. Examples of generic screening criteria include injuries, incidents, documentation failures (including informed consent), failure to respond to abnormal laboratory or X-ray findings, and nosocomial (hospital-acquired) infections. Many of the criteria which define adverse patient occurrences (APOs) are generic.

occurrence screening The process of examining medical records and other data in the hospital (or other health care settings) in order to find cases in which there may have been adverse patient occurrences (APOs), cases which meet predefined criteria. The cases detected by the screening are reviewed by experienced personnel who make judgments as to whether each case should enter the occurrence reporting process for further review. This is a step in the Medical Management Analysis (MMA) system employed by some hospitals in quality management.

screening (diagnostic) Giving diagnostic tests to "normal" individuals or a population in order to detect diseases. The tests employed include examinations of the blood and urine, X-rays, blood pressure measurements, height and weight, questionnaires, and vision and hearing testing. Screening may be employed for detection of a single problem, such as hypertension (high blood pressure) or drug usage, or it may be a "broad spectrum" screening for "anything abnormal" which can be suspected by using a battery of tests. The latter approach is called multiphasic screening (see below).
　　Increasing attention is being given to the cost-benefit ratios of various screening approaches. In a population with very little tuberculosis, for example, the cost of finding new cases by chest X-ray screening is far higher than finding cases by examining contacts of known cases; consequently, chest X-rays are rarely included today in community screening programs. On the other hand, automation of blood chemical determinations has made it often cheaper to perform the standard battery of tests provided by the analyzer than to single out specific tests (which are included in the battery). The laboratory work done in routine examinations on admission to the hospital is primarily a screening process. For example, even though the physician may be most interested in the patient's blood sugar, the whole array of tests—which screens for other disorders—is done simultaneously. Furthermore, such screening on admission to the hospital provides a clinical database on the patient which often helps in timing the onset of abnormalities.

multiphasic screening   Applying batteries of diagnostic tests, usually to persons "on the street" (primarily adults without symptoms) in such settings as shopping malls and county fairs.   Often the tests include some blood chemistry determinations (such as for sugar and cholesterol levels), hearing, blood pressure, intra-eyeball pressure (for detection of glaucoma), and chest X-rays.   The process has been criticized as to its value, on account of such problems as cost per case identified, false positive findings, false negative findings, and unnecessarily alarming the persons tested.

SDM   See *shared decision making.*

second opinion   A consultation which involves the examination of a patient by a surgeon, and the rendering of an opinion by that surgeon, with respect to the need for elective (non-emergency) surgery which has been recommended by another surgeon.

second opinion program   A mandatory or voluntary program calling for second opinions for elective (non-emergency) surgery prior to authorization of the performance of the surgery.

secondary care   Specialized care provided by a physician or hospital, usually on referral from a primary care physician.   Synonym(s): specialized care.

Section 1122   A section of the Social Security Act which denies payment for certain capital expenditures not approved by state planning agencies.

self-care   Those activities that individuals initiate and perform for themselves in connection with their health and well-being.

self-governance   A term commonly used in connection with the medical staff, to which the hospital governing body delegates certain duties, for example, those connected with evaluation of care or the control of physician practices.   It should be noted, however, that the governing body retains the ultimate responsibility for the care in the hospital, even where the medical staff is described as "self-governing."

self-insurance   See *self-insurance* under *insurance.*

self-pay patient   See *self-responsible patient.*

self-referral (patient)   When a patient directly contacts a specialist to obtain secondary care.   This is distinguished from a primary care physician (PCP) making the referral on behalf of the patient.

self-referral (physician)   A physician referring a patient so as to create a conflict of interest.   Physicians are prohibited by federal law from accepting payments from any provider resulting from the referral of Medicare or Medicaid patients.   See also *antikickback law, fraud and abuse,* and *safe harbor regulations.*

self-regulatory entity   See *medical self-regulatory entity.*

self-responsible patient   A patient who pays either all or part of the hospital bill from his or her own resources, as opposed to third-party payment (payment by an insurance company, Medicare, or Blue Cross/Blue Shield (BC/BS)), for example). Synonym(s): self-pay patient.

Senior Plan Network (SPN)   An alliance of health maintenance organizations (HMOs) which offers enrollment in the SPN, and thus in its constituent HMOs. Medicare prepays part or all the cost of enrollment in an SPN as it does in an HMO under certain circumstances.

separate billing   See *separate billing* under *billing*.

service   The term "service" has many meanings in health care, and must always be interpreted in context.

In *health care financing*, a service (or a procedure) is a thing which the payer pays for. Service here means something "done" for a patient by a physician or other person. In medicine, the term "procedure" *also* means something done for a patient. In fact, it is sometimes difficult if not impossible to distinguish the two, since a specific act might equally well be called a "procedure" or a "service. "There are some general guidelines: procedures tend to be distinct actions, and carried out in a brief time as, for example, a surgical operation (a procedure or group of procedures); services (such as preoperative and postoperative care) are less distinct and are carried out over longer (and variable) periods of time. The real answer to what is a service or procedure in financing is whatever the system used by the payer says it is. For physician services, the guide is the *Physician's Current Procedural Terminology (CPT)*. In *CPT*, for example, the physician's "initial hospital care" of a patient is called a "service," although it is largely limited (in billing for care) to what is done upon admission of the patient; each subsequent day's care is defined as another "service." However, the "50-minute hour" in the psychiatrist's office for "medical psychotherapy" is listed as a "procedure. "For purposes of payment, a "service" (or procedure) might more accurately be defined as "the unit for which a charge is made."

Hospitals sometimes use service to refer to a division of the hospital organization, such a the nursing service, or of its medical staff, such as the oncology service. Hospitals also use it for major functions: nursing service, food service, pharmacy, medical records, laboratory, and diagnostic radiology. Hospitals as well as other health care institutions mean support service when they say service; for example, purchasing, maintenance, supplies. These services support the activities of other departments. Hospital services are typically directed by a specific individual who is responsible for its execution, but it may be provided from one central point ("centralized service") or from a number of points in the organization ("decentralized service").

The *marketing* department will use the term service broadly to describe a variety of facilities, programs, and capabilities which provide for various needs of patients and the community. For example, a hospital may provide open heart surgery, genetic counseling, hemodialysis, organ transplants, psychiatric intensive care, weight loss programs, blood pressure screening, and so forth. Each of these might be described as a service.

The American Hospital Association uses service *to classify hospitals* as general or specialized and, if specialized, the nature of the specialty. For example, a hospital's classification according to service could be "children's general hospital" or "alcoholism and other chemical dependency" hospital. A given hospital can be put in only one class according to service.

In *economics*, service means the supplying or meeting of some public demand, as contrasted with producing goods. The health care industry is a "service" industry.

service area The geographic area served by a hospital or other facility or, perhaps more accurately, the area from which the institution or organization draws its patients or clients. A "service area" is sometimes referred to as a "catchment area." The catchment areas of organizations with like services may overlap.

service benefits See *service benefits* under *benefits*.

service contract See *service contract* under *contract*.

settlement An agreement made by the parties to end a dispute or lawsuit before (or during) the hearing or trial, without a formal adjudication (decision by the arbitrator, judge, jury, or other decisionmaker) of the merits of the dispute. The term "settlement" is also sometimes used to refer to the specific terms of the agreement (such as the amount of money to be paid).

structured settlement A settlement which provides for payment of money by the defendant to the plaintiff in other than one lump sum. A structured settlement often provides that the defendant may pay an agreed-upon amount in installments over a period of time. In some cases, a structured settlement might provide that the defendant will reimburse the plaintiff for medical and other expenses as they occur, rather than pay a fixed amount. Other variations are possible, since the terms of the structured settlement are negotiated by the parties.

severity of illness The gravity of a patient's condition. Patients with the same diagnosis often vary from being mildly ill to being extremely ill, or even dying. Under the prospective payment system (PPS), every patient with the same diagnosis (actually, every patient within a given diagnosis related group (DRG), of which there are only 468) is given the same "price tag." No allowance is made for the severity of the patient's illness. Efforts are underway to persuade the federal government to make such an allowance, and other efforts are being made to develop practical methods for quantifying "severity of illness" so that it can be reliably incorporated in the mathematics of the pricing formula. Such quantification is referred to as developing a "severity index" or "score." The stimulus for severity measures is illustrated, for example, by the fact that a diabetic patient in coma (very severely ill) understandably should cost more to treat than one hospitalized simply to "fine-tune" the control of the diabetes. Note that a measure of severity on admission to the hospital, followed by another later measure, permits evaluation of the patient's progress under care, while a measure which can only show severity on discharge does not permit this interpretation.

Several systems are now in development or use in hospitals: Apache II, staging (diseases), patient management categories (PMCs), computerized severity index (CSI), personal computer stager (PC-stager), and MedisGroups.

severity-refined diagnosis related group (SRDRG)   A modified classification system reportedly being readied by the Health Care Financing Administration (HCFA) for use in the Medicare payment process for early implementation. The purpose is to address the criticism of DRGs that they result in the same pay for all patients within a given category, that they do not reflect the fact that some patients are sicker than others, and thus require more resources.

severity score   A mathematical score which expresses the severity of illness of a patient according to one of several severity measurement methods. The goal is to use such scores in a formula for determining payment for care, and in quantifying the quality of care.

shared decision making (SDM)   A growing process in medical care in which physician and patient collaborate in making the decisions as to diagnostic efforts to be made to determine the causes of the patient's problem(s) and the treatments to be used. This sharing of responsibility in SDM results in replacing the authoritarian role traditionally given to the physician with one of consultation and advice, and the passive role of the patient with an active role. Adjustments are required by both physician and patient, as are new tools. See *patient empowerment*.

shared service organization   An organization, external to the hospital, set up to provide shared services, such as group purchasing. Such an organization may or may not have been set up by the organizations receiving the services, and may or may not be under their joint control.

shared services   Administrative, clinical, or other services provided by or for two or more institutions. The services are used jointly or under some arrangement which improves service, reduces cost, or both. A common type of shared service is group purchasing. Synonym(s): cooperative services.

silent PPO   A situation in which insurers cite a PPO discount rate on the explanation of benefits form for patients who do not belong to the PPO.

single-payer plan   A method of health care financing in which there is only one source of money for paying health care providers. The Canadian-style system is the prime example of a single-payer plan, but not all elements of the Canadian program need be included for a plan to be "single-payer"; in fact, the single-payer could be an insurance company. Or the scope of the plan would not have to be national; it could be employed by a single state or community. Proponents of a single-payer plan emphasize the administrative simplicity for patients and providers, and the resulting significant savings in cost.

skilled nursing services   A Medicare term referring to nursing and to other rehabilitation services provided to Medicare beneficiaries under conditions set up by the Medicare program.

smart card   A card which stores in magnetic or optical form information about a patient which can be read by an electronic device. The typical storage medium is a magnetic strip. In general, there are two applications of this technology in health care:
  (1) Personal identification cards similar to credit cards.
  (2) Carrying the individual's medical record. Credit card sized patient cards are

on the market, for example, which, using optical storage technology, can carry 40-80 megabytes of data, i.e., the entire content of a large medical record, including not only text but also images and sound.

snail mail   A nickname for the postal service used to contrast it with e-mail, which travels at electronic speed.

specialty   A particular branch of medicine, or a limited division of another profession, such as nursing. The practitioner of a specialty is a specialist, usually qualified by added training, plus added experience, within the branch of the discipline.

spell of illness   A term, used in determining Medicare benefits, which is defined as a period of time starting when the patient enters the hospital and ending at the conclusion of a 60-consecutive-day period during which the patient has not been an inpatient of any hospital or skilled nursing facility (SNF). (The patient's actual illness ordinarily would have started prior to the hospitalization, and might or might not have concluded within the 60-day period outside the hospital.)

squeal rule   A law requiring a family planning agency to report to parents when family planning advice or services are provided to a minor.

SSI   See *Supplemental Security Income.*

staging (diseases)   One of the methods developed for taking into account a patient's severity of illness, in addition to simply the diagnosis and surgical procedures, in predicting and analyzing the length of stay, cost, and outcome. For a number of diagnoses, objective factors have been identified by which the patient's condition can be classified into several "stages" representing degrees of severity. For example, a diabetic person whose diabetes is under control could be in "Stage 1," and not require hospitalization, while one in diabetic coma (a life-threatening condition) could be in "Stage 4," and require intensive care in the hospital. In this system, the severity score is specific to the disease. As currently applied, using discharge abstract (see *abstract*) data, only the severity on discharge from the hospital can be estimated. Synonym(s): disease staging.

stakeholder   An individual who has an interest in the activities of an organization and the ability to influence it. A hospital's stakeholders, for example, include its patients, employees, medical staff, government, insurers, industry, and the community.

standard of care (medical)   The principles and practices which have been accepted by a health care profession as expected to be applied for a patient under ordinary circumstances. Standards of care are developed from a consensus of experts, based on specific research (where such is available) and expert experience. "Under ordinary circumstances" refers to the fact that a given patient may have individual conditions which are overriding; absent such considerations, a medical staff or nursing staff quality review committee will expect the generally accepted principles and practices to be carried out.

For example, the standard of care for a bedfast patient requires the nursing service to carry out certain procedures to minimize the patient's chances of developing bedsores. The standard of care for a patient with a suspected fracture is to X-ray the area; however, severe bleeding may override (for an extended period of time) the standard calling for the X-ray. In other words, the *first* standard of care is that the individual patient's needs come before the "general" standard. See also *guidelines*.

divided standard of medical care   A proposal by E. Haavi Morreim and others that the "standard of medical care" should be divided into two components: the standard of medical expertise (SME) and the standard of resource use (SRU) in order to distinguish between that which physicians are expected to do for their patients and the resources, monetary and technological, that insurers and others owe to provide to their wards. This divided standard concept is based on the argument that, while physicians throughout the United States have essentially equal access to training and knowledge, and thus could, in general, be held to one SME, the availability of resources is quite a different matter, and the SRU depends on what care or coverage the patient has, and what facilities and other resources are available.

standard of medical expertise (SME)   The standard of care for physicians which measures performance against national norms of training, knowledge, and practice.

standard of resource use (SRU)   A proposed standard of care for a health care provider which measures the resources used in the care of the patient against national norms of use of the same kind and amount of resources. For example, the treatment options available to one physician in an affluent area may not be available to another physician, due to lack of funding or payment, lack of technology, state laws, and so forth. The argument is that a physician should not be held liable for resource inadequacies for which the physician is not responsible.

standard of care (legal)   The measure to be applied, in a malpractice suit, to the actions of the health care professional in order to determine if the professional was negligent. The rule for determining the standard varies from state to state, but it can be generally stated that the standard of care for health care professionals is to exercise that degree of care and skill practiced by other professionals of similar skill and training (and, in some states, in the same geographic locality) under similar circumstances.

The legal "standard of care" may or may not be the same as the medical standard of care in a particular case. The jury (or, in some cases, the judge) in a malpractice case decides what the appropriate "degree of care and skill" is in *that* case, based on the facts and upon the expert testimony offered by both the plaintiff and the defendant. Differences in juries' opinions on the relevant standard of care is one reason why two malpractice cases with similar facts can have different results.

On rare occasions, the legal standard of care may be higher than that of the health care profession. For example, a 32 year old woman developed glaucoma and suffered permanent eye damage, after her physicians failed to detect the condition while treating her from 1959 until 1968. Medical experts for both plaintiff (the woman) and defendant ophthalmologists testified that the standards of the ophthalmology profession did not require routine glaucoma testing for patients under 40. However, the court concluded that since the test was simple, inexpensive, and painless, the standard itself was negligent. *Helling v. Carey*, 83 Wash.2d 514, 519 P.2d 981 (1974).

standard operating procedure (SOP)   An action (or series of actions) to be carried out in a given situation. SOP may or may not be written. For example, it is "SOP" in most households to lock the doors at night.

standardization   A statistical procedure for permitting valid comparisons among several populations. The procedure involves adjustments so that the rates of occurrence of some variable (a disease, for example, by age and sex) are applied to a "standard" distribution of persons by age and sex. Standardization is basically an application of weighting of averages.

stat   "Do at once."

state mandate   See *state mandate* under *mandate*.

statistic   A number calculated from data.

statute   A law enacted (passed) by a legislative body.

statute of limitations   A law requiring that certain types of lawsuits be initiated within a specific length of time. For example, if a patient wishes to sue for malpractice, state law may require that the suit be started within two years after the date of the alleged act of malpractice (the length of time varies from state to state). In some states, the time period begins when the patient discovers (or should have discovered) the injury, rather than on the date of the alleged act of malpractice; this is called the "discovery rule."

In certain circumstances, the law allows the statute of limitations to be suspended ("tolled"). For example, a minor is not legally competent to file suit. Therefore, the law allows that minor to reach majority before the time period begins to run. Thus, even though a statute of limitations for malpractice may be only two years, a suit could be initiated as long as 20 years after the birth of an injured infant (18 years to reach majority, plus the two-year limitations period).

stone center   A lithotripsy facility.

stop-loss insurance   See *stop-loss insurance* under *insurance*.

strategy   A term derived from the military, and which concerns the long-range, large goals of the organization. In traditional thinking, strategy should precede the development of the tactics with which it is implemented. A current insight is that a successful strategy can only be developed after the available tactics are assessed and used to their maximum.

Structured Query Language (SQL)   A computer language for database management, usually pronounced as "sequel" or "S.Q.L". It is probably the most commonly used data management language in the mid 1990's, largely due to its maturity and standardization across varying computer platforms, from microcomputers to mainframes. The language itself, such as "SELECT lastname FROM providers WHERE specialty = 'Surgery'", is often hidden from users by using front end programs which give the user a fill-in-the-form type of interface. SQL was invented by IBM in the 1970's, and ironically, was actually called SEQUEL in its early years. The American National Standards Institute (ANSI) and International Standards Organization (ISO) published an official standard for SQL in 1986, and significantly expanded it in 1992. Additionally, SQL is a US Federal Information Processing Standard (FIPS), which makes it a requirement for many government computer contracts. See also *Online Analytical Processing (OLAP)*.

subacute care   A transitional level of care between acute care and traditional skilled nursing or home care. In some states, subacute care is provided in skilled nursing facility beds.

subscriber   As used in health insurance and with prepayment plans, the subscriber is the person (the eligible employee, for example) who signs up and pays the premiums. Dependents of the subscriber, as well as the subscriber her or himself, are all enrollees (sometimes called members or "covered persons"), but not all enrollees are subscribers.

substance abuse facility   A hospital or other facility specializing in the treatment of patients suffering from alcoholism or chemical dependency.

suicide   Acting in a way which brings about one's own death.

monopoly suicide   An economic phenomenon referring to the observation that any monopoly enterprise which succeeds in raising its prices to the point where "windfall" profits occur will attract such competition into the field that the monopoly will be destroyed.

Supplemental Security Income (SSI)   A federal income support program for low-income aged, blind, and disabled individuals.

support group   A group of individuals with the same or similar problems who meet periodically to share experiences, problems, and solutions, in order to support each other. For example, group members may themselves have, or have a family member or friend suffering from, a disease such as cancer, Alzheimer's, or alcoholism. The group may be sponsored by the individual members, a health care institution, a church, or other body.

SUPPORT Prognostic Model   A system (model) for developing objective estimates of the probable survival over a 180-day period of seriously ill hospitalized adults. The acronym comes from the name of the study which developed the method: "Study to Understand Prognoses and Preferences for Outcomes and Risks of Treatment". The model uses each patient's diagnosis, age, number of days in the hospital before study entry, presence of cancer, neurologic function, and 11 physiologic variables recorded on day 3 after study entry. The study reports that this relatively small number of readily available items of information can provide as good estimates of the probability of survival for 180 days as could physician's estimates. Somewhat better predictions resulted from combining both the objective predictions with physicians'.

Symposium on Computer Applications in Medical Care (SCAMC)   An   annual meeting under the auspices of the American Medical Informatics Association (AMIA).

symptom   A disturbance of appearance or function or sensation of which the patient is or could be aware.   If the disturbance can only be detected by the physician or other observer, it is called a "sign."   Those disturbances which must be elicited by laboratory, X-ray, or other diagnostic procedures, or by response to therapy, are called "findings."

symptom complex   A group of symptoms which occur together, and which may or may not be characteristic of a specific disease.

syndrome   A pattern of signs and symptoms which occur together and form a picture of a given disease.

system (anatomical)   One of the functional components of the body, for example, the respiratory (breathing) system or the circulatory (heart and blood vessels) system.

system (economic)   See *economic system*.

system (process)   A process by which a complex of people and machines (and other essential resources) work together in an orderly fashion to accomplish a given task.

systemic   A term which, in referring to a disease, means a disease that affects the body as a whole.

systems analysis   An analysis of the resources (personnel, facilities, equipment, materials, funds, and other elements), organization, administration, procedures, and policies needed to carry out a given task.   The analysis typically addresses alternatives in each category, and their relative efficiency and effectiveness.

systems review   The traditional method of organizing the medical record under headings such as "respiratory," "past illnesses," or "cardiac."   A newer method, the problem oriented medical record (POMR), instead traces each of the patient's problems separately.

T

tactics   A term derived from the military usage concerning actions which, while directed toward the large goal, are smaller in scale or scope than strategic actions. Tactics are those actions through which a "strategy" is carried out.   Strategy is long-range, and lays out the nature and sequence of the steps to be taken to achieve the large goals of the organization.   In traditional thinking, strategy should precede the development of the tactics with which it is implemented.   A current insight is that a successful strategy can only be developed after the available tactics are assessed and used to their maximum.

tailgate pricing   A pejorative term used to describe pricing which the commentator feels simply responds to the demand of the market (competition) at the moment, that is, pricing which is not based on costs or a consistent pricing policy.

Task Force on National Health Reform   The body created by President Clinton in January 1993, chaired by Hillary Rodham Clinton, with the charge to "listen to all parties and prepare health care reform legislation . . ." It reported that in its deliberations it met with health care providers, consumers, business, and labor groups, including physician groups, nurses groups, hospitals, medical colleges, seniors, long-term care groups, groups representing the disability community, groups specializing in mental health issues, women's groups, children's advocacy groups, minority organizations, rural groups, groups representing small and large businesses, and labor organizations. One of its products was a volume: *Health Care Update: The Need for Health Care Reform.* This was the basis for the health care reform proposal, the Health Security Act, introduced by the President in 1993.

task force   A group of persons established to carry out a specific task. Its assignment is usually fact-finding or advisory. A time limit is typically given by the appointing authority for completion of the task, and upon its completion the task force is automatically disbanded. A task force is not to be confused with a committee, which is a standing body, or a quality circle, which selects its own tasks.

tax credit   An amount that can be subtracted from the tax owed by an individual. Some health care reform proposals include tax credits. These save the individual more money than would the same amount taken as a tax deduction. In some cases, the credit may only reduce the amount of tax owed; in other cases, the credit may actually be refunded to the taxpayer.

tax-deductible   An adjective applied to contributions to 501(c)(3) corporations. The contribution may be taken as a tax deduction by the donor; the term does not refer to the receiving corporation.

tax deduction   An amount which can be subtracted from the taxable income of an individual. Some health care reform proposals include tax deductions as a way to help the individual finance health care. Tax deductions save the individual less money than would the same amount taken as a tax credit.

Tax Equity and Fiscal Responsibility Act (TEFRA)   A 1982 federal act which, among other things, permitted HCFA to enter into risk contracts with HMOs and CMPs, to pay for hospice care, and to extend coverage for ancillary services. It also prohibited employers from keeping employees ages 65 to 69 from participating in the employer's health plan and requiring them to use Medicare instead.

tax-exempt   A nonprofit organization which is not required to pay certain federal (and/or state) taxes. A tax-exempt organization may also qualify to receive tax-deductible donations; see *501(c)(*) corporation.*

tax incentive   A method of encouraging behavior by providing favorable tax treatment (exemptions, deductions, or credits). The Health Security Act (HSA) (1993) proposed several tax incentives: special treatment for long-term care insurance and services; a tax credit for 50% of the cost ($15,000 maximum) of personal care and assistance services for employed individuals with disabilities; and several incentives for providers to encourage primary care services in a health professional shortage area.

tax preference for health benefits   The way that federal law treats health benefits for employees. They have been treated as tax-deductible business expenses for the employer, rather than taxable income to the employee. This practice results in far lower tax revenue for the government.

technology assessment (TA)   The term applied to the growing science of evaluating the costs and benefits of technologies, such as diagnostic imaging for various medical conditions and different situations, electronic devices, diagnostic screening for specific conditions, surgical procedures, and new drugs.

Technology Assessment Conference (TAC)   One of a series of conferences held by the Office of Medical Applications of Research (OMAR) of the National Institutes of Health (NIH), United States Public Health Service (USPHS) to which are invited experts in a particular medical technology in order to develop, and then publish, consensus papers on the use of that technology.

TEFRA   See *Tax Equity and Fiscal Responsibility Act.*

telecommunications (telecom)   Pertaining to the technical aspects of telephones, computer wiring (intra- and inter-building), intercommunication, radio, paging, and other communications systems and networks (excluding computer networks). Traditionally thought of as dealing with voice communications, an increasing amount of computer data (including faxes and multimedia) now flows over telephone lines, blurring any possible distinctions between voice and data. This trend will continue, particularly with the increasing use of ISDN (digital) telephone lines.   See also *National Information Infrastructure (NII).*

telemedicine   Medical care provided through telecommunication when the patient and the caregiver are at separate physical locations. Involves application of interactive audio-visual technology in patient care and education of physicians and other health care personnel, as well as the more traditional access to medical and related records.

telementoring   See *telemedicine.*

telepathology   A technique for sending the image seen through a microscope over a distance to a television monitor. A television camera records the image, which is then transmitted by wire or radio to a remote site where the pathologist can examine the image as though she were looking directly through the viewing microscope. The microscope must be a special, robotically controlled device, so that the pathologist at the remote location can move the slide about and examine various areas, vary the magnification, change the brightness, introduce optical filters, and focus, just as though she were actually seated at an optical microscope.

   This new technique makes possible a number of advances in the quality of care, including providing pathology services to isolated areas, consultations, and instant second opinions. Further possibilities include the use of the technique in the examination of entire organs as well as microscopic sections.

terminal care   Care for a patient in the terminal stages of her illness; care for a dying patient.

tertiary care   Care of a highly technical and specialized nature, provided in a medical center (usually one affiliated with a university), for patients with unusually severe, complex, or uncommon problems. Tertiary care is the highest level of care.

The Medical Directive   See *The Medical Directive* under *advance directive*.

therapeutic   Pertaining to therapy (treatment).

therapy   Treatment. A term which, when used alone, as in "the patient is undergoing therapy," means that the patient is being treated. When used with a modifier, as in "speech therapy," the term means a specific treatment method or technique.

third party   A term used in connection with health care financing. The first and second parties are the patient and the provider. The third party is a payer who is neither of these. Examples are Blue Cross and Blue Shield, commercial insurance, and government. Third parties are increasingly employers, who try to save the money paid to insurance companies or other third parties.

third party administrator (TPA)   An organization which administers health care benefits (and other employee benefits), primarily for corporations which are self-insured. The third party administrator's services include claims review and claims processing, primarily of medical claims but also dental, disability, workers' compensation, life insurance, and pension claims.

third party payer   See *third party payer* under *payer*.

Time Dollar   The term used for local, tax-exempt barter currency in a concept initiated by Edgar Cahn. Individuals participating in a Time Dollar program earn Time Dollars by helping others. One Time Dollar is earned for each hour of volunteer service. A Time Dollar bank account is maintained formally for each participant, and it may be drawn upon by the participant for services by other participants. Also called service credits.

tissue bank   A facility for collecting, cataloging, storing, and distributing body tissues for use in surgery. Bone, for example, is a commonly stored tissue. While the term "tissue" may cover entire organs, organs ordinarily are immediately transplanted rather than banked. The tissues stored in a tissue bank are primarily human. As implantation and transplantation technology advance, an increasing variety of tissues may be expected to be banked, rather than being available only by immediate transfer from donor to recipient. A concomitant development in health care has been the establishment of regional (and national and international) communications networks which help bring together available tissues (and organs) and people who need them.

Title XIX   See *Medicaid*.

Title XVIII   See *Medicare*.

TLC   Tender, loving care.

Tools for Change   A service of the American Hospital Association (AHA) for its members.

tort reform   A change in the way in which individuals who are "harmed" by the health care system may be compensated. In the U.S., patients injured through malpractice or otherwise generally file a lawsuit seeking damages; such suits themselves cost a great deal, take up a lot of time and resources, and may result in enormous sums to the patient. It has been suggested that alternatives might be more fair, result in faster (and often more useful) settlements, and save money. Tort reform is sometimes, in the health care context, referred to as "malpractice reform," although it is not necessarily limited to malpractice cases. See also *alternative dispute resolution (ADR)*, *patients' compensation* (under *compensation*), and *enterprise liability* (under *liability (legal)*).

total quality management (TQM)   See *total quality management (TQM)* under *quality management*.

TQM   See *total quality management (TQM)* under *quality management*.

transitional care   A term covering care which is not acute care and not long-term care. "Transitional care" includes care in postacute convalescence, rehabilitation, and psychiatric care, whether given within acute or long-term care facilities, or in separate programs or facilities.

transplant   To move one living part of the body to another, or from one individual (the "donor") to another. The organ or tissue transplanted is called an "allograft" if from a donor, and an "autograft" (or "homograft") if from the same individual. The term "transplant" may also be used as a noun to indicate the tissue or organ which is transplanted. Synonym(s): graft. See also *implant*.

trauma   A wound or injury. Although one can speak, properly, of psychic trauma, the term in health care usage ordinarily refers to physical injury. Thus "trauma centers" are set up to care for victims of accidents and other violence.

treatment   A term which, when used in "treatment of the patient," means any or all elements of the care of the patient for the correction or relief of the patient's problem. When used in a phrase such as "antibiotic treatment," the term means a specific method or technique. Also called therapy, and sometimes designated with the shorthand notation "Rx."

> **extraordinary treatment**   Medical treatment or care which does not offer a reasonable hope of benefit to the patient, or which cannot be accomplished without excessive pain, expense, or other great burden. The decision whether to provide extraordinary treatment is basically an ethical determination; also, whether treatment is "extraordinary" can only be determined in relation to the condition of the patient and the prognosis. See *futile care*.

triage   Sorting or classification of patients according to the nature and urgency of their illnesses or injuries, and assigning priorities for treatment.

Tringa   A sandpiper, from the Greek "tryngas." In the genus Tringa Linnaeus there are three birds: the greater yellowlegs, the lesser yellowlegs, and the solitary sandpiper. There are, however, 17 other sandpipers which are not in this genus.

trustee   A member of the governing body when that body is called a board of trustees. When the governing body is called the board of directors, then each member is called a "director."

tying arrangement   Requiring a buyer to purchase a second product or service in order to get the first product. Tying arrangements may violate the federal antitrust laws. Synonym(s): tie-in sale.

U

UBIT   See *unrelated business income tax.*

UCR   Usual, customary and reasonable (charge). See *customary, prevailing, and reasonable (CPR).*

ultra vires   "Outside the powers." A legal term referring to activities of a corporation which it is not authorized to do either by its charter or the laws of the state in which it is incorporated.

ultrasound   Sound with a pitch above human hearing (above 20,000 Hz). Ultrasound is used in an imaging technique to visualize internal structures by recording the reflection of the sound waves by the tissues. Ultrasound is also used in some forms of therapy, such as the liquidizing of cataracts and their removal by suction, a process called "phacoemulsufication."

ultrasound images   Images (pictures) of internal body structures, produced by recording (via computer) the sounds wave reflected from the body structures.

umbrella coverage   See *umbrella coverage* under *insurance coverage.*

unbundling   Selling individual components of a service or product separately rather than as a package. Sometimes unbundling is done for the convenience of the customer, but often it is done in order to sell the same components for a greater total price than if they were packaged together (bundled). For example, a complete automobile can be purchased for far less than its parts. In health care, the care of a fracture, for example, may be priced to include the diagnosis, treatment, and aftercare as single package (bundled); alternatively, diagnosis, setting of the fracture, applying the cast, removing the cast, and other services may be priced individually (unbundled).

uncompensated care   Care for which no payment is expected or no charge is made.

under-coding   Submission of a patient's bill with diagnosis or operation coding which will result in a smaller reimbursement than the patient's condition and the care rendered would actually justify. Computer systems which are intended to prevent this are commercially available to health care providers. Compare to over-coding and optimal coding .

underwriting Assuming a risk. In finance, it means assuming the risk of buying a new issue of securities directly from a corporation or government entity, and then reselling them to the public. In insurance, it means assuming the risk of loss in exchange for an amount of money (the premium).

negotiated underwriting A private sale of bonds by their issuer as contrasted with advertisement for public bids. Most hospital bond underwritings are negotiated because of special marketing considerations.

uniform benefit package See *standard benefit package* under *benefit package*.

Uniform Clinical Data Set (UCDS) See *Uniform Clinical Data Set (UCDS)* under *data set*.

Uniform Hospital Discharge Data Set (UHDDS) See *Uniform Hospital Discharge Data Set (UHDDS)* under *data set*.

uniform reporting Reporting of patient care information, financial information, or both under uniform definitions (and sometimes formats) in order to permit comparisons among hospitals or physicians.

unit record A medical record (file) in which are kept the records of all hospitalizations of the individual. This is the preferred method of filing of medical records.

United Network for Organ Sharing (UNOS) A national organ transplant network. This network is under contract to the Health Care Financing Administration (HCFA) to coordinate United States organ procurement activities.

United States Pharmacopeia Convention (USPC) An organization of 325 authorities in medicine, pharmacy, and allied sciences, which revises and publishes the Pharmacopeia of the United States of America (USP) and the National Formulary.

universal coverage, universal insurance coverage See *coverage*.

universal precautions (UP) See *universal precautions* under *precautions*.

Universal Resource Locator (URL) The official name for a site or address of a resource on the Internet. Resources include home pages, graphic images, text files, and digitized sights and sounds (such as movies).

unrelated business income tax (UBIT) Tax paid by a nonprofit corporation on the profits of activities which are not related to the nonprofit purpose of the corporation. A nonprofit corporation is normally exempt from taxation, but may engage in profit-making activities and pay taxes on those, while preserving its tax-exempt status, by complying with specific federal tax law requirements regarding unrelated business income.

UP See *universal precautions* under *precautions*.

upcoding Changing the coding of a patient's diagnoses (and perhaps operations) in order to obtain a higher payment for the services rendered. More accurately called "upclassifying". See also *over-coding*, *under-coding*, and *optimal coding*.

upload   See *download.*

urgent   A term that, in regard to a patient's condition, refers to a degree of illness which is less severe than an emergency, but which requires care within a reasonably short time (more quickly than elective care).

urgent care center   A sort of competitor of an emergency department, but presumably for less "emergent" problems.   The term has no legal (or regulatory) definition as yet.   Sometimes it is stated that a facility, to be called an "urgent care center," must have certain laboratory and X-ray services, but must not hold itself out as ready for emergencies such as those brought by ambulance or to provide continuity of care. An urgent care center may be free-standing or a part of another facility.

Usenet   An Internet (The Net) resource consisting of many online discussion forums about topics ranging from the mundane to the sublime, occasionally prompting some to include ridiculous to the description of topics discussed.   Because of the high volume involved, not all Internet service providers choose to make all forums available to their subscribers.   Forum messages travel over the Net via "newsfeeds", and users participate in the forums via a connection to the Net and the use of software called "newsreaders".

usual, customary and reasonable (UCR)   See *customary, prevailing, and reasonable (CPR).*

utilization review (UR)   See *utilization review* under *review.*

utilization review committee (UR committee)   A committee, made up primarily of medical staff members, designated to carry out the utilization review function, that is, reviewing the appropriateness of hospitalizations and of the services used, and the lengths of stay of patients subject to such review.

V

value-added tax (VAT)   A tax imposed on goods and services at each stage of production.   The end result is similar to a sales tax, but usually produces much more revenue because the tax is not so "visible" and therefore less painful.   It has been discussed as one method of financing health care under health care reform.

value driven   A term being used in health care to categorize a system which has been designed to achieve specified goals in the health of a community and its health care rather than to make financial profit.   Of course, financial profit is also a value, and systems designed to make profits, could also be called value driven.

value history   See *value history* under *advance directive.*

value inventory   A statement elicited from an individual as to that person's values with regard to living and functioning, for example, the person's tolerance for discomfort and pain, desire for personal mobility, willingness to be kept on life support systems, and similar matters. Value inventory questionnaires have been developed as adjuncts to advance directives to make those documents more likely to conform with the individual's own preferences.

vector In public health, a blood-feeding insect, such as a mosquito, which transmits disease.

Veteran's Administration (VA) The federal agency responsible for administering health care programs and facilities for U.S. military veterans. See *Civilian Health and Medical Program of the Uniformed Services (CHAMPUS)* and *Civilian Health and Medical Program of the Veterans Administration (CHAMPVA)*.

viable (can live) Capable of living, as a baby born above a certain birth weight.

viable (can succeed) Capable of being carried out or of succeeding, for example, "viable plans."

virtual community A social aggregation of individuals who develop personal relationships because of their common use of computer mediated communications (CMC), that is, they have become acquainted and continue their association in cyberspace. Such communities appear after the participants carry on discussions over periods of time and discover that they have common interests. Members of a virtual community have no bond other than their interest in the topics of their discussions. Virtual communities are not formed because of geographic, political, or any of the other boundaries which have previously defined communities. Yet they are *real*, and often lead to meetings, picnics, personal associations, and acts of mutual support. Members have carried out fund raising for a community member in need, met and married, and sent flowers for weddings and funerals.

virtual organization An arrangement among actual organizations (or some of their parts) and individuals which carries out functions as though they were provided by a single organization, although the arrangement is not a separate organization. Some emerging health care networks or their programs are virtual organizations. For example, some communities handle teen-aged pregnancy problems with physicians, the local hospital, the local health department, social welfare agencies, churches, and schools each providing some services, working together *seamlessly* as though the "teen-age pregnancy" program were provided by a single organization.

virtual reality An artificial environment created entirely by computer-driven special effects. Virtual reality in modern usage goes well beyond the wearing of special glasses to watch a 3D movie. Not only does virtual reality now create the impression that the environment is real, but it allows one to interact with the artificial environment through use of special equipment. By wearing a special visor and gloves, or even a complete body-suit, the user can simulate the sensation of moving around in the environment. Powerful computer software displays the perspective-corrected images on the visor that create the necessary illusion for the wearer. Sounds and other stimulii may be added to enhance the effect. With computing power becoming ever more economical, there promises to be an explosion in the use of virtual reality. While its entertainment potential certainly gets the most attention, virtual reality already makes it possible to train pilots more safely and economically, and allows the dissection of a frog without a drop of blood ever being spilled.

visit In ordinary use a "visit" means, for example, the appearance of a patient in the emergency department or the appearance of a physician at the bedside. In health care, however, very specific definitions of "visit" are employed in calculation of statistics and in payment. Nevertheless, the use of the term "visit" is not uniform: the "visit" of a patient to an outpatient department in which a physician sees the patient, and then the patient goes to the laboratory and X-ray departments, may be considered one visit or three. Such definitions are often unique to the hospital, the departments involved, and the payment system; one must inquire as to exactly what is meant locally.

office visit All services provided a patient in the course of a single appearance for care at a physician's office.

outpatient visit (OP visit) All services provided an outpatient in the course of a single appearance for care.

visiting nurse association (VNA) A private nonprofit organization with the purpose of providing skilled nursing care and other health care services, primarily in the home, on an hourly basis. Most VNAs are classified as home health agencies.

vital signs A medical term referring to the patient's evidence of heart beat, breathing, and blood pressure. Synonym(s): life signs.

vital statistics Statistics dealing with births, deaths, marriages, and divorces, compiled from official registrations of these events.

voluntary hospital system The national aggregate of nonprofit hospitals and for-profit hospitals in the United States. As in the case of the term "American Hospital System," the voluntary hospital system is not a formal system, but a de facto one.

volunteer A person who performs services without pay. In the hospital, governing body members are often volunteers, as are persons who provide patient assistance services, as well as amenities and revenue-producing services such as the library and gift shop.

voucher A certificate which may be exchanged for a contract for care for a given period of time under a prepayment plan.

voucher system A system in which Medicare beneficiaries use vouchers issued by the federal government to enroll in health care plans of their choice. Early in 1985 Congress enacted legislation permitting this approach to the provision of care for Medicare beneficiaries in an effort to introduce competition into the provision of health care. Under the voucher system, the beneficiary enrolls in a federally qualified health care plan, and payment is made directly to the care-providing organization in a predetermined, fixed amount in exchange for the beneficiary's voucher. Thus, the beneficiary decides which competing health care provider she believes will give the best services (best quality, cheapest, most accessible, or with the most desirable amenities, for example) in exchange for the voucher. The beneficiary receives the services by enrolling in a health care plan, which might be a health care organization (HCO), a health maintenance organization (HMO), a competitive medical plan (CMP), or some other organization set up to provide all the care benefits (outpatient, hospital, home care, and so on) required of a qualified program.

W

---

wage index   See *wage index* under *index (numerical)*.

waiver   A special permission. In health care, a common usage is exemption of a state from participating in the Medicare program under the prospective payment system (PPS) when the state has presented an alternate method of payment which the government has accepted. Similarly, Oregon has been granted a waiver of compliance with regulations as written so that it may use the Oregon plan. States sometimes grant waivers to hospitals to permit special usage of allied health professionals in order to permit implementation of innovative methods of health care delivery.

weighting   A statistical method for combining numerical data from more than one source into a single value. Each value from a given source is usually multiplied by a factor (its "weight") which has been judged by the person producing the statistic to represent the importance of that factor in relation to the importance of the other factors going into the single final value. A simple example of the importance of weighting is found when it is necessary to "average averages" (it is usually stated that "you must NOT average averages"). For example, if a group of people was made up of 100 women with average height of 5 feet and 200 men with average height of 6 feet, it would be incorrect to simply add the two averages and divide by 2 (since there are two values going into the total): $5+6/2=5.5$ feet (5'6"). "The correct method is one of weighting: $5 \times 100 + 6 \times 200 = 1200$. Then 1200 is divided by 300 (total persons). The weighted average is 5.66 feet (5'8").

well-baby care   Health care services to normal babies in order to detect any problems early and to give preventive advice. This is the counterpart of prenatal care for pregnant women.

well-year   The equivalent of one completely well year of life, a measure designed to assess the benefits of health programs. The measure is used in a General Health Policy Model (GHPM). The well-year value is derived from measures of (1) life expectancy and (2) health-related quality of life (HRQOL) during years before death. If an individual, for example, was judged to be functioning at a 60% level (as rated on the investigator's scale) for one year, he would be considered to have had 0.60 well-years of life.

Whole Earth 'Lectronic Link (WELL)   One of the earliest citizen-operated computer conferencing systems which enable people around the world to carry on public conversations and exchange private electronic mail (e-mail). The WELL was developed by the publishers of the Whole Earth Catalog in 1985.

wholistic health   See *holistic health*.

wide area network (WAN)   Two or more local area networks (LANs) connected together, typically over telephone lines or satellite links. In an university, for example, each department usually has its own LAN. These LANs are connected together throughout the university to form a WAN for the entire campus. The transmission medium connecting the LANs together is called a "backbone", and the information traffic among the LANs is handled by a special computer called a "router". WANs can, of course, also be connected together, also with the aid of a router.

withhold   The portion of a payment due a physician in a managed care plan which is held back by the plan in order to provide a contingency fund to be used in case 1) the usage under the plan exceeds the predictions under which the premiums were established, and the plan is unable to pay the full amount (the withheld money is needed for more claims or other unexpected costs), and 2) in case the plan has a system for releasing the withhold variably to different physicians under a formula which takes into account the relative productivity and performance of each physician. The withheld amount is typically about 20% of the claims, and is sometimes called the "physician contingency reserve" (PCR).

Women, Infants, and Children's Program (WIC)   A federally funded program which provides specific food vouchers and nutrition education to "at risk" pregnant women and children five years old and under.

workers' compensation (WC)   See *workers' compensation (WC)* under *compensation*.

World Health Organization (WHO)   The division of the United Nations (UN) which is concerned with health.

wraparound coverage   See *wraparound coverage* under *insurance coverage*.

X

xenograft   An organ or tissue implanted (grafted) from one species to another. The Baby Fae case, in which the heart of a baboon was transplanted into a human baby, was a case in which a xenograft was used. Synonym(s): heterograft.

Z

ZEBRA   See *Zero Balanced Reimbursement Account.*

Zero Balanced Reimbursement Account (ZEBRA)   A type of health care benefit plan provided by employers who are self-insured and pay for the care as it is given. The ceiling under such a plan is typically "unlimited." The Internal Revenue Service (IRS) has ruled that funds spent for a beneficiary (here an employee) under such a plan are taxable to the beneficiary, and that the employer is liable for withholding income tax on benefits, except for those benefits which are nontaxable under federal statutes. Distinguished from cafeteria plans because a ZEBRA does not qualify under Section 125 of the IRS Code.

Notes

Notes

Ordering Information

For over ten years, Tringa Press has been providing guidance through the maze of jargon of health care and other disciplines.

Responding first to the need of laypersons -- such as new hospital trustees -- we soon learned that the need was far wider, because so many terms, proliferating daily, were not defined *anywhere*.

Health Care Terms, THIRD COMPREHENSIVE EDITION
By Vergil N. Slee, Debora A. Slee, & H. Joachim Schmidt
Softbound, approx. 700 pages, April 1996, $49.95, Order No. HCT3

In five years, *Health Care Terms, Comprehensive Edition* has more than doubled in content -- over 5,000 terms defined! And, new features include appendices containing an overview of current health care issues, U.S. and abroad; a table of health care delivery organizations; and a special "how to find out what you can't find out here (or anywhere else)" section.

Health Care Terms, HEALTHY COMMUNITIES EDITION
By Vergil N. Slee, Debora A. Slee, & H. Joachim Schmidt
Softbound, approx. 208 pages, January 1996, $19.95, Order No. HC1

Order directly from Tringa Press. To make books accessible to trustees, students, and other groups, we offer substantial quantity discounts: 20% for 5-19 copies; 40% for 20 or more. We also pay the shipping costs on prepaid orders.

Please send:

____copies of Health Care Terms, *Third Comprehensive Edition* @ $49.95

____copies of Health Care Terms, *Healthy Communities Edition* @ $19.95

S & H (if not prepaid): 1-4 books $4; 5-19 books $7; 20 or more $10.

Name _____

Title _____

Institution _____

Address _____

City, State, Zip _____

Phone/Fax_____

Tringa Press, P.O. Box 8181, St. Paul, MN 55108
612-222-7476; FAX 612-699-0666; help@tringa.com
http://www.tringa.com